Rorschachiana 43

Rorschachiana

Journal of the International
Society for the Rorschach

Volume 43 / Issues 1&2 / 2022

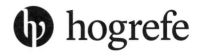

Editorial Assistant	Arianna Antonelli, Italy
Responsible Organization	International Society of the Rorschach and Projective Methods (ISR) https://www.internationalrorschachsociety.com/ Treasurer Tanja Franjkovic, c/o Hogrefe AG, Länggass-Str. 76, 3012 Bern, Switzerland
Current President of ISR	Fernando Silberstein
Past Presidents of ISR	Marguerite Loosli-Usteri, Robert Heiss, Adolf Friedemann, Kenowar Bash, Nina Rausch de Traubenberg, John Exner, Irving Weiner, Anne Andronikof, Bruce L. Smith, Noriko Nakamura
Publication	Rorschachiana is available as a book and as a journal (consisting of two online issues per year, an annual print compendium, and online access to back issues): ISBN 978-0-88937-629-8 (Rorschachiana, Vol. 43) ISSN 1192-5604 (journal)

Rorschachiana, Volume 43, 2022 (Book)

Publishing Offices   USA: Hogrefe Publishing Corporation, 44 Merrimac Street, Suite 207, Newburyport, MA 01950
Phone +1 978 255-3700, E-mail customersupport@hogrefe.com
EUROPE: Hogrefe Publishing GmbH, Merkelstr. 3, 37085 Göttingen, Germany
Phone +49 551 99950-0, Fax +49 551 99950-111; E-mail publishing@hogrefe.com

Sales and   USA: Hogrefe Publishing, Customer Services Department,
Distribution   30 Amberwood Parkway, Ashland, OH 44805, Phone (800) 228-3749,
Fax (419) 281-6883; E-mail customersupport@hogrefe.com
UK: Hogrefe Publishing, c/o Marston Book Services Ltd., 160 Eastern Ave.,
Milton Park, Abingdon, OX14 4SB, Phone +44 1235 465577,
Fax +44 1235 465556; E-mail direct.orders@marston.co.uk
EUROPE: Hogrefe Publishing, Merkelstr. 3, 37085 Göttingen, Germany
Phone +49 551 99950-0, Fax +49 551 99950-111;
E-mail publishing@hogrefe.com

Other Offices   CANADA: Hogrefe Publishing, 82 Laird Drive, East York, Ontario, M4G 3V1
SWITZERLAND: Hogrefe Publishing, Länggass-Strasse 76, 3012 Bern

Printed and bound in the Czech Republic

ISBN   978-0-88937-629-8

Rorschachiana: Journal of the International Society for the Rorschach

Publisher   Hogrefe Publishing GmbH, Merkelstr. 3, 37085 Göttingen, Germany,
Phone +49 551 99950-0, Fax +49 551 99950-111, publishing@hogrefe.com
USA: Hogrefe Publishing Corporation, 44 Merrimac Street,
Suite 207, Newburyport, MA 01950, USA, Phone +1 978 255-3700,
E-mail customersupport@hogrefe.com

Production   Juliane Munson, Hogrefe Publishing, Merkelstr. 3, 37085 Göttingen, Germany,
Phone +49 551 99950-422, Fax +49 551 99950-111, production@hogrefe.com

Subscriptions   Hogrefe Publishing, Herbert-Quandt-Str. 4, 37081 Göttingen, Germany,
Phone +49 551 99950-900, Fax +49 551 99950-998,
journalsdistribution@hogrefe.com

Advertising / Inserts   Hogrefe Publishing, Merkelstr. 3, 37085 Göttingen, Germany,
Phone +49 551 99950-423, Fax +49 551 99950-111, marketing@hogrefe.com

ISSN   1192-5604

Publication   Published in two online issues and a print compendium per annual volume.

Subscription Prices   Calendar year subscriptions only. Rates for 2023: Institutions - from US $259.00/
€221.00 (detailed pricing can be found in the journals catalog at hgf.io/journals
catalog); Individuals - US $143.00/€106.00 (print & online). Single issue (online
only) - US $135.00/€118.00

Payment   Payment may be made by check, international money order, or credit card, to
Hogrefe Publishing, Merkelstr. 3, 37085 Göttingen, Germany. US and Canadian
subscriptions can also be ordered from Hogrefe Publishing, 44 Merrimac Street,
Suite 207, Newburyport, MA 01950, USA

Electronic Full Text   The full text of *Rorschachiana* is available online at www.econtent.hogrefe.com

Abstracting Services   Abstracted/indexed in PsycINFO, PSYNDEX, Scopus, EMCare, and Cinahl
Information Systems.

The Rorschach® Test has probably generated more subsequent literature in the field of psychology than any other work. Due to its universal applicability, timeless appeal to clinicians, and proven track record, this particular instrument has been utilized many millions of times throughout the world.

For more than 60 years, the International Society of the Rorschach and Projective Methods has played an important role in promoting the research and application of the Rorschach and other projective techniques. The first Congress of the Society took place in Zurich in August 1949. Subsequent meetings have been held periodically through the years, in a variety of locations: Rome (1956), Brussels (1958), Freiburg (1961), Paris (1965), London (1968), Zaragosa (1971), Fribourg (1977), Washington (1981), Barcelona (1984), Guarujá, São Paulo (1987), Paris (1990), Lisbon (1993), Boston (1996), Amsterdam (1999), Rome (2002), Barcelona (2005), Leuven / Louvain (2008), Tokyo (2011), Istanbul (2014), and Paris (2017). The ISR Centenary Congress was held in Geneva, Switzerland, in 2022.

To contribute to *Rorschachiana,* authors are welcome to submit papers:

1) targeting the metrics and the validity of any of the Rorschach systems available in literature with the goal of providing users with more reliable, sensitive, and useful procedures to administer and interpret the test;
2) focusing on the understanding of the client's perception of projective measures within online testing practices;
3) that provide visibility to all projective measures, especially those with demonstrated reliability and validity, and show their clinical utility to understand and help clients;
4) on new tests, or new coding systems for traditional tests, providing scientifically sound literature reviews of these measures, illustrating the psychometric properties of their coding systems, demonstrating their clinical utility, and informing readers about the training procedures available to become proficient in their use.

Contents

Volume 43, Issue 1, 2022

Volume 43, Issue 2, 2022

Special Issue: New Insights From Other Psychological Disciplines for Rorschach Users

Research Article

The Effects of Subliminal Emotional Priming on Rorschach Responses

Luciano Giromini[1], Sharon Carfora Lettieri[1], Jessica Bosi[2], and Alessandro Zennaro[1]

[1]Department of Psychology, University of Turin, Italy
[2]Department of Psychology, University of Surrey, Guilford, UK

Abstract: The Rorschach is one of the most popular performance-based tests and it is thought to provide information on relatively stable individual differences, including respondent inclinations and preferences. To investigate the extent to which minor, nonconscious, emotional fluctuations in the respondent's mind could influence Rorschach scores, we used a backward masking paradigm. More specifically, each Rorschach card was presented on a computer screen twice, once under a neutral and once under an emotional priming condition. In the neutral priming condition, the target stimulus of the backward masking procedure was a neutral face; in the emotional priming condition, the target stimulus of the backward masking procedure was an angry face. A sample of 182 healthy, adult volunteers contributed to this study. Statistical analyses revealed that Rorschach scores obtained from the neutral versus emotional conditions were similar to each other.

Keywords: Rorschach, priming, emotion, subliminal, backward masking

The Rorschach (Rorschach, 1921) is one of the most popular performance-based tests and it shows how an individual responds to the question "What might this be?" when exposed to 10 inkblot designs. Based on how the test-takers explore the visual stimuli, what content(s) they see, what about the inkblot made them see what they saw, what themes they describe, how well they communicate what they saw, and many other behavioral features, the assessor obtains a very unique overall picture of the test-takers' psychological functioning (Meyer & Eblin, 2012). Despite it being almost 100 years old, the Rorschach is still taught and used widely: over 60% of American doctoral programs teach it (Mihura et al., 2017) and over 50% of practitioners claim to use it as an assessment tool (Wright et al., 2017).

An evidence-based method that is growing in popularity is the Rorschach Performance Assessment System (R-PAS; Meyer et al., 2011). It was developed to let the predominant method of evaluating the Rorschach, the Comprehensive System (CS; Exner, 2003), continue to evolve after the death of its creator. It is largely based on the findings of a recent series of meta-analyses that examined 65 main variables in the CS and found that some variables had stronger validity (particularly those that target cognitive and perceptual processes) compared to others (Mihura et al., 2013). Additionally, the selection of variables to include in R-PAS was based on the relationship between the presumed response-process behind a code and its associated interpretation, as well as on a worldwide survey of clinicians on the utility of various CS variables (Meyer et al., 2011). As a result, 60 R-PAS Summary Scores are now organized into Page 1 and Page 2 Profiles, with variables on Page 1 being interpretatively more important and more supported psychometrically. It should be noted that although R-PAS builds on and significantly extends the research endeavors initiated by the CS, it differs in many ways, so that it can be considered an independent and – for many – psychometrically improved alternative to that method.

The Rorschach is deemed to investigate traits, individual inclinations, and preferences as opposed to temporary states. This is supported by research suggesting that nearly all the CS variables associated with trait characteristics show stability in adults over long periods of time (Sultan et al., 2006), and that lower stability is primarily related with only diffuse shading (Y) and inanimate movement (m), which are considered to be sensitive to state variations (Exner, 2003; Viglione & Hilsenroth, 2001; Weiner, 2001). To date, however, very few studies have investigated whether *minor* fluctuations in psychological states influence Rorschach scores.

A relatively widely used approach to induce small variations in mental and emotional states involves exploiting the phenomena of attentional or sensory unawareness (Tamietto & de Gelder, 2010). In relation to the former, when an individual is completely unaware of *emotional* information, threat information is prioritized even when it is task-irrelevant (even when individuals are told to ignore it) and therefore can still affect attention (Hedger et al., 2016; Norberg et al., 2010). Regarding the latter, nonconsciously perceived emotional stimuli can elicit physiological responses as well as generate facial muscle movement mirroring the emotion conveyed by the stimulus (Dimberg et al., 2000; Tamietto et al., 2009). Both of these processes have been investigated using numerous priming paradigms including dual-task, binocular rivalry and backward masking (Tamietto & de Gelder, 2010). Briefly, a dual-task paradigm involves presenting two tasks or stimuli, each with different goals, simultaneously or in quick succession, often resulting in a performance disruption in the more cognitively demanding of the two. Binocular rivalry paradigms involve the simultaneous presentation of different images to the eyes. One image dominates perception and is consciously perceived whereas the other is suppressed, due to the alternate inhibition of monocular channels in the primary visual cortex. In a backward masking paradigm, an emotional target stimulus is presented momentarily (typically < 30 ms), immediately followed by a neutral "masking" stimulus so that the participant is unaware of the first stimulus and only reports the neutral one (Esteves et al., 1994; Whalen et al., 1998). Typically, priming from masked stimuli has been shown to only have very brief psychological, motivational, and physiological effects, lasting from mere fractions of a second to a maximum of a few seconds (Wentura & Rothermund, 2014).

There is a very limited number of studies exploring the impact of *priming* and emotional inducement on Rorschach responses. On conducting a search on PsycINFO for "Rorschach" and "priming" with linked full text, three were found but only one was relevant to this research. In this study, students were primed with three short videos with nonemotive content (people tossing balls to each other) aimed at activating the mirror neuron system (MNS) at different levels, and immediately after they were administered Rorschach cards (Giromini, Viglione, et al., 2016). The impact was slight, but the sample size was very small with a limited number of responses (three responses to three cards), so that the generalizability of these findings might be questioned.

One further study of this kind was presented recently at a Society of Personality Assessment (SPA) conference in which participants completed the Rorschach immediately after viewing violent or sad film content for 2-3 min (Hsiao et al., 2019). Participants (N = 37) who watched the aggressive scene had elevated Rorschach scores across multiple domains (including Aggressive Movement [AGM], Morbid Content [MOR], and Aggressive Content [AGC]) compared to controls (N = 66), suggesting that Rorschach responses might be sensitive to temporary psychological states induced by viewing emotive material. It should be noted, however, that because the content of the videos was rather explicit, one cannot rule out the possibility that participants' responses were not only influenced by their emotions but also because they anticipated the goal of the study or they tended to simply remember the content of the videos (which is evidently different from responding based on emotional fluctuations). In terms of predicting the aim of the study, participants may have been explicitly or implicitly induced to "please" the experimenter based on what they believed the experimenter expected from them, as it is known that some of the aforementioned variables (e.g., AGC, AGM, etc.) can easily be manipulated by the respondent (Benjestorf et al., 2013). Therefore, the design of this research does not clarify whether Rorschach responses are indeed influenced by the induced emotional state of the participant and leaves open the possibility that there are other reasons for the response variations. To that extent, using a backward masking paradigm could be beneficial because research participants might be influenced by the stimuli without being aware of it.

The goal of the current study was to test the impact of temporary emotional fluctuations on Rorschach responses and scores. To do so, we relied on a backward masking paradigm as described earlier. Cards were presented after showing two different series of stimuli, one beginning with an emotionally loaded image shown for 10 ms, the other beginning with a neutral image shown for 10 ms. The aim was to test whether nonconsciously induced emotional states would influence Rorschach responding. Additionally, we also tested whether individual differences on emotional regulation and intelligence would moderate the impact of those emotional fluctuations on Rorschach responding.

On the basis of the aforementioned literature, we expected emotional subliminal priming to have minimal influence on Rorschach responding except perhaps for individuals with weaker emotion regulation skills. The Rorschach variables that we expected to be more strongly influenced by emotional subliminal priming were those theoretically associated with anger (e.g., AGM and AGC), because the emotionally loaded images used to generate emotional priming were angry faces (see next section).

Before starting this study, the research project was reviewed by the Institutional Review Board (IRB) of the University of Turin, Italy, and approved on September 21, 2017 (protocol no. 348369). All procedures were indeed in accordance with the ethical standards of the institutional and national research committee and with the 1964 Helsinki Declaration and its later amendments or comparable ethical standards.

Method

Participants

The initial sample consisted of 186 participants (female $n = 131$, male $n = 52$, other $n = 3$) ranging in age from 18 to 73 ($M_{age} = 30.19$, $SD = 11.75$, unreported age $n = 3$). The majority were single, students or nonclinical participants from the community (i.e., 170). Four participants' data, however, were ultimately excluded from the analyses as more than 10% of the items of their emotional dysregulation- or intelligence-related questionnaires (see next section) were left unanswered. Thus, the final sample comprised 182 adult volunteers.

To take part, participants had to have no prior knowledge of the Rorschach, be aged 18 or older, be clinically healthy with no clinically relevant disorders (i.e., not be receiving any form of psychiatric or psychotropic treatment), and be able to read Italian. Anybody with a psychiatric diagnosis or neurological issue, history of drug or alcohol abuse or use of psychotropic drugs, and pregnant women or women who were breastfeeding were excluded from participating. Informed consent was given by all participants.

Measures

The Karolinska Directed Emotional Faces (KDEF; Lundqvist et al., 1998)
The KDEF is a set of 490 color images of human facial expressions, containing pictures of 70 individuals (35 males and 35 females ranging in age from 20 to 30 years) exhibiting seven emotional expressions (angry, happy, sad, neutral, surprised, fearful, and disgusted). Each expression is viewed from five angles and was recorded twice. The KDEF is a widely used, validated instrument (Goeleven et al., 2008). A sample of 60 Caucasian faces (15 men and 15 women) was used in this study, either portraying anger or a neutral emotion. Angry faces have been tested before in this context and have been shown to have an impact on psychophysiological reactions (Tamietto et al., 2009; Tamietto & de Gelder, 2010).

Difficulties in Emotion Regulation Questionnaire (DERS; Gratz & Roemer, 2004)
The DERS is a widely used, comprehensive 36-item self-report measure of six facets of subjective emotion-regulation abilities: (1) awareness and understanding of emotion, (2) clarity of emotion, (3) acceptance of one's emotions, (4) ability to adopt efficient and effective regulation strategies, (5) capability to adopt goal-directed behaviors, and (6) ability to manage impulses when experiencing negative emotions. Individuals must select a rating from a scale of 1 (*almost never*) to 5 (*almost always*), and item responses are added together to calculate a total DERS score as well as six subscale scores. Higher scores indicate greater difficulties in emotion regulation. A shorter, 16-item version of the DERS, introduced and validated by Bjureberg and colleagues in 2016, was used in this study (Bjureberg et al., 2016).

We speculated that individuals with decreased emotional regulation abilities could be more vulnerable to small emotional fluctuations and therefore could be more influenced by the subliminal priming. Thus, we used the DERS to test whether emotional regulation difficulties could moderate the impact that the priming had on participants' Rorschach responding processes. To maximize power, we only focused on the total DERS score and did not look at the subscale scores.

The Italian version adapted by Giromini et al. (2012) was used in this study as its factorial structure has adequately replicated the six-factor structure and, overall, its scores have demonstrated good validity as well as test–retest reliability (Giromini et al., 2012). More specifically, we extracted from the original Italian version of the DERS the 16-item identified by Bjureberg and colleagues (2016) in order to obtain an Italian version of the DERS-16. In this study, Cronbach α was .91 for the total DERS-16 score.

Trait Meta-Mood Scale (TMMS; Salovey et al., 1995)

The TMMS is a 30-item self-report scale designed to understand and evaluate individual differences in people's ability to attend and react to their moods and changes in them. It consists of three subscales: Attention, a subscale that refers to the subjectively observed attention given to one's own emotional states (e.g., "I pay a lot of attention to how I feel"); Clarity, a subscale that evaluates one's understanding of their own emotional state (e.g., "I am rarely confused about how I feel"); and Repair, a subscale that informs on the perceived ability to regulate emotions and mood states (e.g., "Although I am sometimes sad, I have a mostly optimistic outlook"). Individuals must evaluate their level of agreement with each statement on a 5-point Likert scale ranging from 1 = *totally disagree* to 5 = *totally agree*. It is one of the most widely used and most useful instruments to assess differences in the reflective mood experience (Fernández-Berrocal & Extremera, 2008).

In addition to emotional dysregulation, emotional intelligence as measured by the TMMS could also serve as a moderator of the impact of subliminal priming on Rorschach responding, as we anticipated that more emotionally intelligent individuals would possibly be less vulnerable to small emotional fluctuations. Also in this case, we focused on the total score, rather than on the subscale scores, in order to maximize statistical power. The adapted and validated Italian version of the TMMS was used (Giromini et al., 2017). Cronbach's α, in this study, was .85 for the total TMMS score.

Procedure

A snowball convenience sample was recruited via email, social networking, word of mouth, and posters in the Psychology Department at the University of Turin. An email address was provided if individuals wished to volunteer to take part in the study. Data collection took place over a 2-year period from 2017 to 2019.

A suitable time and date were arranged with participants to visit the Psychology Department where they first completed demographic information followed by the TMMS and DERS. The Rorschach was then administered using a response phase that required some adjustments. A backward masking procedure (see Figure 1) was used before presenting each Rorschach card. More specifically, in the neutral condition, a neutral face from the KDEF was first displayed for 10 ms, then a set

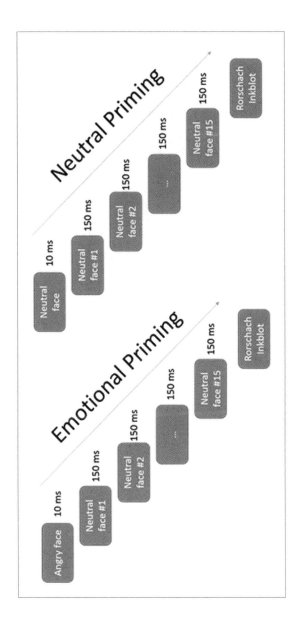

Figure 1. In the neutral condition, a neutral face was first displayed for 10 ms; then a set of 15 neutral faces were presented for 150 ms each; finally, the Rorschach inkblot was presented. In the emotional priming condition, the neutral face lasting for 10 ms was substituted with an angry face; then, the same neutral faces used in the neutral condition were used, prior to presenting the Rorschach inkblot. For each Rorschach card, participants delivered two responses: one in the neutral priming condition, one in the emotional priming condition. The order of presentation of the two conditions (i.e., emotional vs. neutral priming) was randomized and counterbalanced. Thus, each participant produced 20 responses (2 per card), 10 following neutral priming and 10 following emotional priming.

of 15 neutral faces – also from the KDEF – were presented for 150 ms each (for a total of 2,250 ms), and, finally, the Rorschach inkblot was presented. In the emotional priming condition, the neutral face lasting for 10 ms was substituted with an angry face, which also was taken from the KDEF; then the same neutral faces used in the neutral condition were used, prior to presenting the Rorschach card. Each participant completed 20 responses, 10 following neutral priming and 10 following emotional priming. The order of presentation of the two conditions (i.e., neutral and emotional) was randomized and counterbalanced for each card. It should be noted that a pilot testing conducted on a few individuals prior to initiating the study revealed that, as desired, test-takers could not tell the difference between the neutral and emotional priming conditions.

In the response phase, the 10 Rorschach cards were presented on a computer screen, using Presentation and were formatted to be the same size as the printed versions of the cards. For each card, participants were instructed to think of a single response only. After the first exposure, the 10 Rorschach cards were then presented for a second time and participants had to think of one additional response for each card. In accordance with standard R-PAS procedures, during this phase the experimenter sat next to the participant and wrote down all responses verbatim. In the clarification phase, participants were handed printed versions of the Rorschach cards (i.e., the standard Rorschach plates) and asked to clarify their previous responses following standard R-PAS procedures (Meyer et al., 2011).

Participants were debriefed at the end, thanked for their participation, and were given the opportunity to learn more about the experiment.

Reliability Check

To examine interrater reliability, two advanced graduate students independently re-coded 20 of the protocols included in this study, under the supervision of an expert R-PAS user who had been using R-PAS for years. As reported in Tables 1 and 2, intraclass correlation coefficients (ICCs) demonstrated fair-to-excellent interrater reliability (Cicchetti, 1994; Shrout & Fleiss, 1979), consistent with previously published research articles addressing R-PAS interrater reliability (Pignolo et al., 2017; Schneider et al., 2020; Viglione et al., 2012).

Data Analysis

To test the impact of emotional subliminal priming on Rorschach responses, we first calculated the protocol-level R-PAS scores of each participant generated by considering the 10 responses produced following neutral priming and those generated by considering the 10 responses produced following emotional priming. In this step, consistent with previous research (e.g., Pignolo et al., 2017) and R-PAS

Table 1. Main effect of priming on R-PAS summary scores on Page 1

R-PAS variable	ICC	Neutral		Emotional		Main effect of priming		
		M	SD	M	SD	$F_{(1, 179)}$	Uncorrected p	d
Engagement & Cognitive Processing								
Complexity	.97	31.85	8.86	31.16	8.51	0.08	.78	0.08
F%	.95	42.80	20.46	41.96	21.64	0.01	.93	0.04
Blend	.96	1.68	1.59	1.77	1.61	0.18	.67	−0.06
Sy	.86	2.81	1.78	2.64	1.71	0.06	.80	0.09
MC	.93	3.38	1.85	3.40	1.92	1.19	.28	−0.01
MC – PPD	.87	0.14	2.58	0.04	2.56	0.53	.47	0.04
M	.90	1.86	1.30	1.95	1.40	1.12	.29	−0.07
M – WsumC	.84	0.34	1.60	0.50	1.72	0.32	.57	−0.10
CFC – FC	.58	−0.03	1.51	0.04	1.37	0.14	.70	−0.05
Perception & Thinking Problems								
EII-3	.85	−0.20	0.70	−0.20	0.69	0.59	.44	−0.01
TP-Comp	.76	0.80	1.24	0.86	1.26	0.47	.50	−0.04
WSumCog	.89	2.59	4.30	2.51	4.53	0.84	.36	0.05
SevCog	.83	0.10	0.39	0.12	0.48	0.00	.98	−0.04
FQ–%	.65	13.15	12.37	14.01	13.00	1.44	.23	−0.07
WD–%	.64	11.78	11.84	12.73	12.63	0.51	.48	−0.08
FQo%	.89	58.67	16.90	58.03	17.19	0.38	.54	0.04
Popular	.72	2.05	1.24	2.34	1.46	4.98	.03	−0.21
Stress & Distress								
YTVC'	.84	1.64	1.59	1.78	1.61	0.09	.77	−0.09
m	.84	0.55	0.81	0.53	0.76	0.27	.60	0.03
Y	.93	0.58	0.77	0.65	0.87	0.48	.49	−0.08
MOR	.74	0.51	0.78	0.55	0.77	0.23	.63	−0.07
SC-Comp	.85	4.23	0.92	4.22	0.97	0.12	.73	0.02
Self & Other Representation								
ODL%	.67	6.97	9.09	6.80	8.49	1.94	.17	0.02
SR	.49	0.34	0.66	0.37	0.65	0.00	.96	−0.08
MAP – MAH	.72	−0.21	0.77	−0.23	0.75	2.15	.14	0.01
PHR – GHR	.85	−0.93	1.79	−0.88	1.91	0.01	.93	−0.02
M−	.87	0.30	0.56	0.25	0.55	0.45	.51	0.09
AGC	.90	1.23	1.21	1.32	1.26	0.03	.86	−0.07
V-Comp	.87	1.83	0.99	1.72	0.94	0.00	.96	0.12
H	.87	1.45	1.17	1.33	1.19	0.00	.97	0.10
COP	.93	0.66	0.82	0.70	0.93	0.55	.46	−0.04
MAH	.87	0.36	0.63	0.37	0.62	0.46	.50	−0.03

Note. Variables shown in bold were square-root transformed prior to calculating ICC, *F*, *p*, and *d* values. Variables that are italicized are proportion variables computed as subtraction. None of the results is statistically significant after applying Bonferroni–Holm correction.

Table 2. Main effect of priming on R-PAS summary scores on Page 2

R-PAS Variable	ICC	Neutral		Emotional		Main effect of priming		
		M	SD	M	SD	F(1, 179)	Uncorrected p	d
Engagement & Cognitive Processing								
W%	.98	54.13	21.84	54.75	20.27	1.46	.23	−0.03
Dd%	.98	7.48	10.14	7.12	8.87	0.36	.55	0.04
SI	.68	0.97	0.94	0.87	1.05	0.61	.43	0.09
IntCont	.83	0.75	1.32	0.80	1.60	0.01	.92	0.00
Vg%	.93	3.21	6.57	4.28	7.59	1.22	.27	−0.14
V	.86	0.11	0.35	0.17	0.43	1.19	.28	−0.15
FD	.57	0.46	0.71	0.48	0.75	0.06	.81	−0.03
WSumC	.86	1.52	1.14	1.45	1.17	0.14	.71	0.06
C	.69	0.23	0.47	0.28	0.54	0.07	.79	−0.09
Mp − Ma	.49	−0.36	1.46	−0.36	1.48	0.30	.58	0.00
Perception & Thinking Problems								
FQu%	.65	26.98	14.93	26.42	13.53	0.05	.82	0.04
Stress & Distress								
PPD	.92	3.24	2.25	3.36	2.32	0.00	.95	−0.05
CBlend	.62	0.30	0.56	0.27	0.56	4.01	.05	0.08
C'	.49	0.84	1.08	0.81	1.06	0.35	.55	0.03
CritCont%	.85	20.05	17.36	21.16	17.27	0.11	.74	−0.06
Self & Other Representation								
SumH	.97	3.13	1.69	2.97	1.61	0.17	.68	0.10
NPH − H	.69	0.23	1.86	0.31	1.96	0.06	.80	−0.04
refl	1.00	0.18	0.42	0.30	0.53	0.09	.76	−0.27
p − a	.49	−0.82	2.12	−0.72	1.88	1.68	.20	−0.05
AGM	.77	0.23	0.53	0.25	0.56	0.17	.68	−0.06
T	.86	0.10	0.34	0.15	0.41	0.01	.90	−0.14
PER	.70	0.09	0.34	0.06	0.26	0.15	.70	0.11
An	.96	0.75	0.91	0.76	0.91	0.12	.73	−0.01

Note. Variables shown in bold were square-root transformed prior to calculating ICC, *F*, *p*, and *d* values. Variables that are italicized are proportion variables computed as subtraction. None of the results is statistically significant after applying Bonferroni–Holm correction.

guidelines (www.r-pas.org), for R-PAS proportion scores, we computed the difference between the numerator and the second code composing the denominator of the target proportion score. For instance, the variable Passive Movement Proportion, which in R-PAS is obtained by dividing the number of Passive Movement responses by the sum of Active and Passive Movement responses [p/(a + p)], was computed as Passive Movement minus Active Movement [p − a]. Next, we inspected descriptive statistics to check for possible nonnormality issues. A square root transformation was applied to variables with absolute skew values greater than 2 or absolute kurtosis values greater than 7 (see Curran et al., 1996). Finally, we ran a series of ANCOVAs, with priming (neutral vs. emotional) as the within-subject factor, the total DERS and total TMMS scores as covariates, and each of the R-PAS Summary Scores on Page 1 and Page 2 as the dependent variables. Considering the relatively large sample size ($N = 182$), each ANCOVA was supposed to be able to reliably detect a small-to-medium effect size (with power = .80 and $\alpha = .05, f = .209$).

Because the Rorschach stimuli were presented on a computer screen, and given that participants were asked to give exactly one response to each exposure of each card (for a total of two responses per card), R-PAS variables Prompts (Pr), Pulls (Pu), Card Turning (CT), Number of Responses (R), and Eight-Nine-Ten Percent (R8910%) were not analyzed. As such, the total number of R-PAS variables included in the analyses was 55. To account for the multiple testing problem, Bonferroni–Holm correction (considering 55 tests) was adopted to evaluate the statistical significance of results. With regard to the determination of the size of the main effects of priming on Rorschach responding, in line with recommendations by Dunlap et al. (1996), Cohen's d values were calculated using standard independent samples d formula.

Results

Most of the R-PAS variables under investigation, that is, 41, were normally distributed based on the Curran et al. (1996) criterion mentioned earlier (skew ≤ 2.0 and kurtosis ≤ 7.0). For 10 of the remaining 14 variables, a square root transformation was able to normalize the distribution. For Vista (V), Severe Cognitive Codes (SevCog), Texture (T), and Personal Knowledge Justification (PER), we could not find a way to remove the nonnormality problems. As such, in addition to the ANCOVAs presented here, we also performed some nonparametric analyses, which still led to exactly the same conclusions and therefore are not reported.

As shown in Tables 1 and 2, none of the 55 tested main effects was statistically significant after applying Bonferroni–Holm correction. Cohen's d ranged from –.27 (for Reflections; Refl) to .12 (for Vigilance Composite; V-Comp), with the mean of the absolute d values being .07 ($SD = .05$). The effect size values reported here refer to the contrasts between the two priming conditions (neutral vs. emotional), regardless of respondents' scores on DERS and TMMS. By contrast, the F values reported in Tables 1 and 2 refer to the results of ANCOVAs computed using the

DERS and TMMS scores as covariates. This explains why Refl has one of the smallest $F(0.09)$ and largest p values (.76), even though its effect size is larger than that of all other variables. The influence of subliminal priming on R-PAS scores should thus be characterized as null or very small (Cohen, 1988). Furthermore, neither emotional regulation, nor emotional intelligence significantly interacted with the effects of priming (Tables 3 and 4). Also in this case, the size of the inspected interaction effects was extremely small, approximating $\eta_p^2 = 0.00$ for almost all of the summary R-PAS scores on Page 1 or Page 2.

Additional Analyses

Of all Page 1 and Page 2 R-PAS scores, only Popular (P) yielded an uncorrected p lower than .05 when evaluating the main effect of priming ($p = .03$). Although this result did not remain statistically significant after Bonferroni–Holm correction, we wanted to understand in more depth the possible impact of subliminal emotional priming on P responses by adopting a Bayesian approach. Indeed, because classic null-hypothesis significance tests are known to be biased toward rejection, especially when the sample size is relatively large as is in our case (for background, see Berger & Sellke, 1987; Edwards et al., 1963; Goodman, 1999; Rouder et al., 2009; Sellke et al., 2001; Wagenmakers, 2007), we wanted to more directly compare the likelihood that the null versus the alternative hypotheses would be true, given the data. To do so, we relied on Rouder and colleagues' (2009) JZS B, which had already been used in the Rorschach literature before (e.g., Giromini, Viglione, et al., 2015; Reese et al., 2014). Briefly, the Rouder et al. (2009) JZS B allows us to evaluate the ratio of the probability of obtaining our data under the null hypothesis (i.e., the priming has no impact on P) to the probability of obtaining our data under the alternative hypothesis (i.e., the priming does have an impact on P). The results of these additional analyses generated a JZS B of 1.24, which therefore slightly favors the null over the alternative. Said differently, even if we analyzed P only, rather than all 55 selected variables, there would still be no strong evidence that the subliminal emotional priming used in this study had any influence on P responses.

Discussion

The aim of this study was to evaluate the impact of subliminal priming of emotional faces to see whether brief emotional fluctuations influence Rorschach responses. A backward masking task where either a neutral face or angry face was the target stimulus was used and Rorschach responses were compared within

Table 3. Interaction effects of priming with DERS and TMMS on R-PAS summary scores on Page 1

R-PAS variable	Priming × DERS			Priming × TMMS		
	$F(1, 179)$	p	η_p^2	$F(1, 179)$	p	η_p^2
Engagement & Cognitive Processing						
Complexity	0.08	.78	0.01	1.01	.32	0.00
F%	0.01	.93	0.00	0.61	.43	0.00
Blend	0.18	.67	0.00	0.30	.58	0.00
Sy	0.06	.80	0.01	1.36	.25	0.00
MC	1.19	.28	0.00	0.69	.41	0.01
MC – PPD	0.53	.47	0.00	0.20	.66	0.00
M	1.12	.29	0.00	0.59	.44	0.00
M – WSumC	0.32	.57	0.00	0.14	.71	0.00
CFC – FC	0.14	.70	0.00	0.62	.43	0.00
Perception & Thinking Problems						
EII-3	0.59	.44	0.00	0.38	.54	0.00
TP-Comp	0.47	.50	0.00	0.00	.97	0.00
WSumCog	0.84	.36	0.01	1.56	.21	0.00
SevCog	0.00	.98	0.00	0.15	.69	0.00
FQ–%	1.44	.23	0.00	0.25	.62	0.01
WD–%	0.51	.48	0.00	0.11	.74	0.00
FQo%	0.38	.54	0.00	0.20	.65	0.01
Popular	4.98	.03	0.02	4.05	.05	0.02
Stress & Distress						
YTVC'	.09	.77	0.00	0.04	.84	0.00
m	.27	.60	0.00	0.40	.53	0.00
Y	.48	.49	0.01	1.11	.29	0.00
MOR	.23	.63	0.01	1.49	.22	0.01
SC-Comp	.12	.73	0.01	1.16	.28	0.00
Self & Other Representation						
ODL%	1.94	.17	0.00	0.04	.84	0.01
SR	.00	.96	0.01	1.07	.30	0.00
MAP – MAH	2.15	.14	0.01	1.93	.17	0.01
PHR – GHR	.01	.93	0.00	0.00	.96	0.00
M–	.45	.51	0.00	0.46	.50	0.00
AGC	.03	.86	0.01	1.58	.21	0.00
V-Comp	.00	.96	0.00	0.02	.88	0.00
H	.00	.97	0.00	0.55	.46	0.00
COP	.55	.46	0.00	0.14	.71	0.00
MAH	.46	.50	0.00	0.14	.71	0.00

Note. Variables shown in bold were square-root transformed prior to calculating F, p, and η_p^2 values. Variables that are italicized are proportion variables computed as subtraction. None of the results is statistically significant after applying Bonferroni–Holm correction.

Table 4. Interaction effects of priming with DERS and TMMS on R-PAS summary scores on Page 2

R-PAS Variable	Priming × DERS			Priming × TMMS		
	$F(1, 179)$	p	η_p^2	$F(1, 179)$	p	η_p^2
Engagement & Cognitive Processing						
W%	1.46	.23	0.00	0.16	.69	0.01
Dd%	0.36	.55	0.00	0.01	.94	0.00
SI	0.61	.43	0.01	1.54	.22	0.00
IntCont	0.01	.92	0.01	1.06	.30	0.00
Vg%	1.22	.27	0.00	0.80	.37	0.01
V	1.19	.28	0.00	0.54	.46	0.00
FD	0.06	.81	0.02	3.42	.07	0.01
WSumC	0.14	.71	0.00	0.11	.74	0.00
C	0.07	.79	0.00	0.02	.87	0.00
Mp − Ma	0.30	.58	0.00	0.88	.35	0.00
Perception & Thinking Problems						
FQu%	0.05	.82	0.00	0.64	.43	0.00
Stress & Distress						
PPD	.00	.95	0.00	0.01	.92	0.00
CBlend	4.01	.05	0.01	1.60	.21	0.02
C'	.35	.55	0.00	0.52	.47	0.00
CritCont%	.11	.74	0.00	0.69	.41	0.00
Self & Other Representation						
SumH	0.17	.68	0.00	0.24	.63	0.00
NPH − H	0.06	.80	0.00	0.25	.62	0.00
refl	0.09	.76	0.00	0.48	.49	0.00
p − a	1.68	.20	0.02	4.19	.04	0.00
AGM	0.17	.68	0.00	0.02	.90	0.00
T	0.01	.90	0.00	0.53	.47	0.00
PER	0.15	.70	0.00	0.24	.62	0.00
An	0.12	.73	0.00	0.37	.55	0.00

Note. Variables shown in bold were square-root transformed prior to calculating F, p, and η_p^2 values. Variables that are italicized are proportion variables computed as subtraction. None of the results is statistically significant after applying Bonferroni–Holm correction.

subjects between the two conditions. The results provide preliminary evidence to suggest that subliminal emotional priming does not influence R-PAS Summary Scores on either Page 1 or Page 2.

Subliminal priming has been shown to impact decision-making tasks such as the selection of suitable candidates for a job role (Skandrani-Marzouki & Marzouki,

2010) and the buying and consumption of beverages (Winkielman et al., 2005) as well as influencing social behavior such as physically moving away from a group stereotyped as being dangerous or violent (Wyer & Calvini, 2011). Furthermore, it has also been shown to influence social judgments by altering very early perceptual analyses when analyzing event-related potentials (ERP) in the brain, especially the P1 component (Li et al., 2008). Therefore, current evidence suggests that subliminal priming could impact both behavior and neurobiological responses.

Conversely, our results suggest that Rorschach responses are fairly resistant to the intervention used in this study, which other researchers have shown can induce temporary, nonconscious mood changes. Indeed, no significant relationship was found between the R-PAS variables examined and the different priming conditions, even though our sample was relatively large so that power was adequate. In terms of applicative implications, while we always encourage practitioners to attend to all R-PAS guidelines (Meyer et al., 2011) with regard to the administration setting (e.g., to make sure that there are no notable distractions in the room, to investigate the emotional status of the examinee prior to beginning administration, etc.), the results of our study suggest that the presence of minimal implicit stimulations (e.g., a painting eliciting emotional responses, etc.) might not dramatically influence our examinee's performance on the Rorschach task.

The ability to regulate emotions involves being able to effectively manage and respond to an emotional experience, without allowing it to take control over one's behavior (Gross & Thompson, 2007). With this in mind, when we designed this study, we speculated that small, nonconscious mood changes could perhaps have a greater impact on Rorschach responses of more, rather than less, emotionally dysregulated individuals. Contrary to our expectations, what we found is that self-reported levels of emotional intelligence and emotion regulation *did not* moderate the influence that our subliminal priming had on our participants' responses. Arguably, two plausible explanations could account for this nonsignificant finding. First, there is some debate as to whether an individual who lacks emotional intelligence or emotion regulation abilities can accurately measure their own ability to manage their emotions, as emotional awareness is deemed to be a key factor of both emotional intelligence and emotion regulation (e.g., Giromini, Brusadelli, et al., 2015; Gratz & Roemer, 2004; Mayer et al., 2002). To evaluate this possible explanation, future research could attempt to replicate our findings by using a performance-based measure of emotional intelligence such as the Mayer–Salovey–Caruso emotional intelligence test (MSCEIT; Mayer et al., 2002). Second, it is possible that the effect of our subliminal priming was simply too weak to be able to observe any measurable changes in the test-takers' behavior. In other words, it is possible that a floor effect occurred, so that future replications with a more impactful stimulation (e.g., rather than using angry faces, one could try using snakes; Tamietto & de Gelder, 2010) would be beneficial.

Limitations

This study is not without its limitations. Firstly, although extant literature – including a review published in a *Nature* journal (Tamietto & de Gelder, 2010) – suggests that subliminal emotional priming typically influences one's behavioral and psychophysiological reactions (Dimberg et al., 2000; Hedger et al., 2016; Li et al., 2008; Norberg et al., 2010; Wyer & Calvini, 2011), we did not have any tools in our study to measure the extent to which our emotional priming really induced a temporary, nonconscious mood change. To overcome this limitation, future research could consider including the recording of galvanic skin responses (Giromini, Ando', et al., 2016; Porges, 1991; Weems et al., 2005) or a similar indicator. Second, it is possible that because the same emotional stimulus was repeated 10 times for each participant, some habituation occurred. Somewhat relatedly, the fact that we relied exclusively on a relatively specific visual image (i.e., angry faces) to generate emotional priming might call into question the generalizability of our results to other types of visual images and representations. It should be noted, however, that these two limitations characterize most of the studies implementing a backward masking paradigm, which, however, have still shown some observable effects (Tamietto & de Gelder, 2010). Third, the ecological validity of our study might be questioned, given the fact that the Rorschach inkblots were shown on a computer screen, rather than under standard procedures. Furthermore, the lack of a clinical sample did not allow us to test whether participants with severely impaired emotional regulation abilities would show a greater vulnerability to subliminal priming compared with healthy individuals. In addition, our interrater reliability check showed that six of the variables included in the analyses had suboptimal reliability, with ICCs in the range between .40 and .59 (i.e., *fair* interrater reliability, according to Cicchetti, 1994). This may be particularly problematic because these ICCs may have overestimated the reliability of the actual scores used in the data analyses, since they were calculated using all 20 responses from each protocol, whereas the scores examined in the main analyses contained only 10 responses per condition. Finally, although it is known that subliminal priming effects typically do not last longer than a few seconds (Wentura & Rothermund, 2014), we could not measure the actual duration of subliminal priming effects in our experiment. Considering this, another potential flaw in our study is that the emotional priming condition may have lasted longer than expected and affected the response(s) to the following card(s) too, which would introduce some noise and error variance.

Conclusion

Notwithstanding these limitations, the results of our study still suggest that Rorschach responses are likely not susceptible to the effects of subliminal emotional priming, at least as we and others have implemented it, with an angry face shown for an imperceptible 10 ms interval followed by 15 perceivable neutral masks lasting for 2,250 ms. Ultimately, this is good news in relation to Rorschach administration as it suggests that – pending future replications – emotion-inducing incidents occurring before undertaking the Rorschach are likely to have a limited impact on an individual's responses. If replicated – not only with subliminal emotional priming, but also with more explicit and conscious emotional stimuli – this research could possibly support that the Rorschach is a robust assessment tool that can be safely used even immediately following emotional events that are likely to occur in day to day life and that could precede taking the test, such as having an argument with a friend or being late because of a paucity of available parking spots.

References

Benjestorf, S. T., Viglione, D. J., Lamb, J. D., & Giromini, L. (2013). Suppression of aggressive Rorschach responses among violent offenders and nonoffenders. *Journal of Interpersonal Violence, 28*(15), 2981–3003. https://doi.org/10.1177/0886260513488688

Berger, J. O., & Sellke, T. (1987). Testing a point null hypothesis: The irreconcilability of P values and evidence. *Journal of the American Statistical Association, 82*(397), 112–122. https://doi.org/10.1080/01621459.1987.10478397

Bjureberg, J., Ljótsson, B., Tull, M., Hedman, E., Sahlin, H., Lundh, L., Bjärehed, J., DiLillo, D., Messman-Moore, T., Hellner Gumpert, C., & Gratz, K. (2016). Development and validation of a brief version of the difficulties in emotion regulation scale: The DERS-16. *Journal of Psychopathology and Behavioral Assessment, 38*(2), 284–296. https://doi.org/10.1007/s10862-015-9514-x

Cicchetti, D. V. (1994). Guidelines, criteria, and rules of thumb for evaluating normed and standardized assessment instruments in psychology. *Psychological Assessment, 6*(4), 284–290. https://doi.org/10.1037/1040-3590.6.4.284

Cohen, J. (1988). *Statistical power analysis for the behavioral sciences* (2nd ed.). Erlbaum.

Curran, P. J., West, S. G., & Finch, J. F. (1996). The robustness of test statistics to nonnormality and specification error in confirmatory factor analysis. *Psychological Methods, 1*(1), 16–29. https://doi.org/10.1037/1082-989X.1.1.16

Dimberg, U., Thunberg, M., & Elmehed, K. (2000). Unconscious facial reactions to emotional facial expressions. *Psychological Science, 11*(1), s86–s89. https://doi.org/10.1111/1467-9280.00221

Dunlap, W. P., Cortina, J. M., Vaslow, J. B., & Burke, M. J. (1996). Meta-analysis of experiments with matched groups or repeated measures designs. *Psychological Methods, 1*(2), 170–177. https://doi.org/10.1037/1082-989X.1.2.170

Edwards, W., Lindman, H., & Savage, L. J. (1963). Bayesian statistical inference for psychological research. *Psychological Review, 70*(3), 193–242. https://doi.org/10.1037/h0044139

Esteves, F., Dimberg, U., & Ohman, A. (1994). Automatically elicited fear: Conditioned skin conductance responses to masked facial expressions. *Cognition and Emotion, 8*(5), 393–413. https://doi.org/10.1080/02699939408408949

Exner, J. E. J. (2003). *The Rorschach: A comprehensive system: Vol. 1. Basic foundations* (4th ed.). Wiley.

Fernández-Berrocal, P., & Extremera, N. (2008). A review of trait meta-mood research. *International Journal of Psychology Research, 2*, 39–67. https://doi.org/10.1177/0734282914550384.0.94

Giromini, L., Ando', A., Morese, R., Salatino, A., Di Girolamo, M., Viglione, D. J., & Zennaro, A. (2016). Rorschach performance assessment system (R-PAS) and vulnerability to stress: A preliminary study on electrodermal activity during stress. *Psychiatry Research, 246*, 166–172. https://doi.org/10.1016/j.psychres.2016.09.036

Giromini, L., Brusadelli, E., Di Noto, B., Grasso, R., & Lang, M. (2015). Measuring psychological mindedness: Validity, reliability, and relationship with psychopathology of an Italian version of the balanced index of psychological mindedness. *Psychoanalytic Psychotherapy, 29*(1), 70–87. https://doi.org/10.1080/02668734.2015.1006666

Giromini, L., Colombarolli, M. S., Brusadelli, E., & Zennaro, A. (2017). An Italian contribution to the study of the validity and reliability of the trait meta-mood scale. *Journal of Mental Health, 26*(6), 523–529. https://doi.org/10.1080/09638237.2017.1340621

Giromini, L., Velotti, P., de Campora, G., Bonalume, L., & Cesare Zavattini, G. (2012). Cultural adaptation of the difficulties in emotion regulation scale: Reliability and validity of an Italian version. *Journal of Clinical Psychology, 68*(9), 989–1007. https://doi.org/10.1002/jclp.21876

Giromini, L., Viglione, D. J., Brusadelli, E., Zennaro, A., Di Girolamo, M., & Porcelli, P. (2016). The effects of neurological priming on the Rorschach; A pilot experiment on the human movement response. *Rorschachiana, 37*(1), 58–73. https://doi.org/10.1027/1192-5604/a000077

Giromini, L., Viglione, D. J., & McCullaugh, J. (2015). Introducing a Bayesian approach to determining degree of fit with existing Rorschach norms. *Journal of Personality Assessment, 97*(4), 354–363. https://doi.org/10.1080/00223891.2014.959127

Goeleven, E., De Raedt, R., Leyman, L., & Verschuere, B. (2008). The Karolinska directed emotional faces: A validation study. *Cognition & Emotion, 22*(6), 1094–1118. https://doi.org/10.1080/02699930701626582

Goodman, S. N. (1999). Toward evidence-based medical statistics. 2: The Bayes factor. *Annals of Internal Medicine, 130*(12), 1005–1013. https://doi.org/10.7326/0003-4819-130-12-199906150-00019

Gratz, K., & Roemer, L. (2004). Multidimensional assessment of emotion regulation and dysregulation: Development, factor structure, and initial validation of the difficulties in emotion regulation scale. *Journal of Psychopathology and Behavioral Assessment, 26*(1), 41–54. https://doi.org/10.1023/B:JOBA.0000007455.08539.94

Gross, J. J., & Thompson, R. A. (2007). Emotion regulation: Conceptual foundations. In J. J. Gross (Ed.), *Handbook of emotion regulation* (pp. 3–24). Guilford Press.

Hedger, N., Gray, K. L. H., Garner, M., & Adams, W. J. (2016). Are visual threats prioritized without awareness? A critical review and meta-analysis involving 3 behavioral paradigms and 2696 observers. *Psychological Bulletin, 142*(9), 934–968. https://doi.org/10.1037/bul0000054

Hsiao, W., Meyer, G. J., Mihura, J. L., O'Gorman, E. T., & Charek, D. B. (2019). *The effect of induced psychological states on selected Rorschach thematic scores and self-reported experiences.* Unpublished manuscript.

Li, W., Zinbarg, R. E., Boehm, S. G., & Paller, K. A. (2008). Neural and behavioral evidence for affective priming from unconsciously perceived emotional facial expressions and the influence of trait anxiety. *Journal of Cognitive Neuroscience, 20*(1), 95–107. https://doi.org/10.1162/jocn.2008.20006

Lundqvist, D., Flykt, A., & Öhman, A. (1998). *The Karolinska directed emotional Faces – KDEF (CD ROM).* Karolinska Institute, Department of Clinical Neuroscience, Psychology Section.

Mayer, J. D., Salovey, P., & Caruso, D. (2002). *Mayer–Salovey–Caruso emotional Intelligence Test (MSCEIT) user manual.* Multi-Health Systems.

Meyer, G. J., & Eblin, J. (2012). An overview of the Rorschach performance assessment system (R-PAS). *Psychological Injury and Law, 5*(2), 107–121. https://doi.org/10.1007/s12207-012-9130-y

Meyer, G. J., Viglione, D. J., Mihura, J. L., Erard, R. E., & Erdberg, P. (2011). *Rorschach performance assessment system: Administration, coding, interpretation, and technical manual.* Rorschach Performance Assessment System, LLC.

Mihura, J. L., Meyer, G. J., Dumitrascu, N., & Bombel, G. (2013). The validity of individual Rorschach variables: Systematic reviews and meta-analyses of the comprehensive system. *Psychological Bulletin, 139*(3), 548–605. https://doi.org/10.1037/a0029406

Mihura, J. L., Roy, M., & Graceffo, R. A. (2017). Psychological assessment training in clinical psychology doctoral programs. *Journal of Personality Assessment, 99*(2), 153–164. https://doi.org/10.1080/00223891.2016.1201978

Norberg, J., Peira, N., & Wiens, S. (2010). Never mind the spider: Late positive potentials to phobic threat at fixation are unaffected by perceptual load. *Psychophysiology, 47*(6), 1151–1158. https://doi.org/10.1111/j.1469-8986.2010.01019.x

Pignolo, C., Giromini, L., Ando', A., Ghirardello, D., Di Girolamo, M., Ales, F., & Zennaro, A. (2017). An interrater reliability study of Rorschach performance assessment system (R-PAS) raw and complexity-adjusted scores. *Journal of Personality Assessment, 99*(6), 619–625. https://doi.org/10.1080/00223891.2017.1296844

Porges, S. W. (1991). Vagal tone: An autonomic mediator of affect. In *The development of emotion regulation and dysregulation* (pp. 111–128). Cambridge University Press. https://doi.org/10.1017/CBO9780511663963.007

Reese, J. B., Viglione, D. J., & Giromini, L. (2014). A comparison between comprehensive system and an early version of the Rorschach performance assessment system administration with outpatient children and adolescents. *Journal of Personality Assessment, 96*(5), 515–522. https://doi.org/10.1080/00223891.2014.889700

Rorschach, H. (1921). *Psychodiagnostik.* Bircher.

Rouder, J., Speckman, P., Sun, D., Morey, R., & Iverson, G. (2009). Bayesian *t* tests for accepting and rejecting the null hypothesis. *Psychonomic Bulletin & Review, 16*(2), 225–237. https://doi.org/10.3758/PBR.16.2.225

Salovey, P., Mayer, J. D., Goldman, S. L., Turvey, C., & Palfai, T. P. (1995). Emotional attention, clarity, and repair: Exploring emotional intelligence using the trait meta-mood scale. In *Emotion, disclosure, & health* (pp. 125–154). American Psychological Association. https://doi.org/10.1037/10182-006

Schneider, A., Bandeira, D. R., & Meyer, G. J. (2020). Rorschach Performance Assessment System (R-PAS) interrater reliability in a Brazilian adolescent sample and comparisons with three other studies. *Assessment.* Advance online publication. https://doi.org/10.1177/1073191120973075

Sellke, T., Bayarri, M. J., & Berger, J. O. (2001). Calibration of *p* values for testing precise null hypotheses. *The American Statistician, 55*(1), 62–71.

Shrout, P. E., & Fleiss, J. L. (1979). Intraclass correlations: Uses in assessing rater reliability. *Psychological Bulletin, 86*(2), 420–428. https://doi.org/10.1037/0033-2909.86.2.420

Skandrani-Marzouki, I., & Marzouki, Y. (2010). Subliminal emotional priming and decision making in a simulated hiring situation. *Swiss Journal of Psychology/Schweizerische Zeitschrift für Psychologie/Revue Suisse de Psychologie, 69*(4), 213–219. https://doi.org/10.1024/1421-0185/a000025

Sultan, S., Andronikof, A., Réveillère, C., & Lemmel, G. (2006). A Rorschach stability study in a nonpatient adult sample. *Journal of Personality Assessment, 87*(3), 330–348. https://doi.org/10.1207/s15327752jpa8703_13

Tamietto, M., Castelli, L., Vighetti, S., Perozzo, P., Geminiani, G., Weiskrantz, L., & de Gelder, B. (2009). Unseen facial and bodily expressions trigger fast emotional reactions. *Proceedings of the National Academy of Sciences of the United States of America, 106*(42), 17661–17666. https://doi.org/10.1073/pnas.0908994106

Tamietto, M., & de Gelder, B. (2010). Neural bases of the non-conscious perception of emotional signals. *Nature Reviews Neuroscience, 11*(10), 697–709. https://doi.org/10.1038/nrn2889

Viglione, D. J., Blume-Marcovici, A. C., Miller, H. L., Giromini, L., & Meyer, G. (2012). An inter-rater reliability study for the Rorschach performance assessment system. *Journal of Personality Assessment, 94*(6), 607–612. https://doi.org/10.1080/00223891.2012.684118

Viglione, D. J., & Hilsenroth, M. J. (2001). The Rorschach: Facts, fictions, and future. *Psychological Assessment, 13*(4), 452–471. https://doi.org/10.1037/1040-3590.13.4.452

Wagenmakers, E. J. (2007). A practical solution to the pervasive problems of *p* values. *Psychonomic Bulletin & Review, 14*(5), 779–804.

Weems, C. F., Zakem, A. H., Costa, N. M., Cannon, M. F., & Watts, S. E. (2005). Physiological response and childhood anxiety: Association with symptoms of anxiety disorders and cognitive bias. *Journal of Clinical Child & Adolescent Psychology, 34*(4), 712–723. https://doi.org/10.1207/s15374424jccp3404_13

Weiner, I. B. (2001). Advancing the science of psychological assessment: The Rorschach inkblot method as exemplar. *Psychological Assessment, 13*(4), 423–432. https://doi.org/10.1037/1040-3590.13.4.423

Wentura, D., & Rothermund, K. (2014). Priming is not priming is not priming. *Social Cognition, 32*(Suppl), 47–67. https://doi.org/10.1521/soco.2014.32.supp.47

Whalen, P. J., Rauch, S. L., Etcoff, N. L., McInerney, S. C., Lee, M. B., & Jenike, M. A. (1998). Masked presentations of emotional facial expressions modulate amygdala activity without explicit knowledge. *Journal of Neuroscience, 18*(1), 411–418. https://doi.org/10.1523/JNEUROSCI.18-01-00411.1998

Winkielman, P., Berridge, K. C., & Wilbarger, J. L. (2005). Unconscious affective reactions to masked happy versus angry faces influence consumption behavior and judgments of value. *Personality and Social Psychology Bulletin, 31*(1), 121–135. https://doi.org/10.1177/0146167204271309

Wright, C. V., Beattie, S. G., Galper, D. I., Church, A. S., Bufka, L. F., Brabender, V. M., & Smith, B. L. (2017). Assessment practices of professional psychologists: Results of a national survey. *Professional Psychology: Research and Practice, 48*(2), 73–78. https://doi.org/10.1037/pro0000086

Wyer, N. A., & Calvini, G. (2011). Don't sit so close to me: Unconsciously elicited affect automatically provokes social avoidance. *Emotion (Washington, DC), 11*(5), 1230–1234. https://doi.org/10.1037/a0023981

History
Received November 17, 2021
Revision received February 24, 2022
Accepted February 24, 2022
Published online April 28, 2022

Conflict of Interest
The authors declare that they have no conflict of interest.

Publication Ethics
All procedures performed in studies involving human participants were in accordance with the ethical standards of the institutional and/or national research committee and with the 1964 Helsinki Declaration and its later amendments or comparable ethical standards. The Institutional Review Board of University of Turin approved the research project on September 21, 2017 (protocol no. 348369).
Informed consent was obtained from all individual participants included in the study.

Open Data
Authors are willing to share their data set upon reasonable request. To obtain the data set associated with this article, please contact the corresponding author at luciano.giromini@unito.it

ORCID
Luciano Giromini
 https://orcid.org/0000-0002-9540-4803

Luciano Giromini
Department of Psychology
University of Turin
Via Verdi 10
10123 Turin
Italy
luciano.giromini@unito.it

Summary

The effects of emotional priming on Rorschach responses have been poorly studied. In particular, no study to date has examined whether subliminal priming might have an impact on the Rorschach response processes. To address this gap in the literature, we used a backward masking paradigm and tested whether showing the Rorschach inkblot designs after neutral subliminal priming and emotional subliminal priming would elicit different types of responses. Specifically, we recruited a nonclinical sample of 182 adult volunteers and gave them the Difficulties in Emotion Regulation Questionnaire (DERS) and the Trait Meta-Mood Scale (TMMS) to complete. Next, we administered the Rorschach test using the following experimental procedure: Each Rorschach card was presented twice on a computer screen, once under a neutral priming condition and once under an emotional priming condition. In the neutral priming condition, the target stimulus of the backward masking was a neutral face; in the emotional priming condition, the target stimulus of the backward masking was an angry face. In both conditions, the target stimulus remained on the screen for 10 ms, so it could only be processed at a nonconscious level. Participants' responses in the neutral or emotional priming conditions were then scored and compared using the Rorschach Performance Assessment System (R-PAS). In addition, we also wanted to test the hypothesis that individuals with diminished emotional regulation abilities might be more susceptible to small emotional fluctuations and therefore more influenced by subliminal priming. Accordingly, we conducted a series of ANCOVAs with priming (neutral vs. emotional) as a within-subject factor, DERS and TMMS total scores as covariates, and each of the R-PAS Summary Scores on Page 1 and Page 2 as dependent variables. The results showed that the Rorschach scores obtained in the neutral and emotional priming conditions were remarkably similar, regardless of the emotion regulation and emotional intelligence level of the participants. Taken together, these results suggest that subliminal priming is unlikely to affect the Rorschach response process, although other stimuli and research designs are needed to reach such a conclusion.

Riassunto

Gli effetti del priming emotivo sulle risposte al test di Rorschach sono stati poco studiati in letteratura. In particolare, nessuno studio fino ad oggi ha esaminato se il priming di tipo subliminale possa avere un impatto sui processi di risposta al Rorschach. Per colmare questa lacuna della letteratura, abbiamo utilizzato un paradigma di *backward masking* e abbiamo testato se presentare le macchie di Rorschach dopo stimoli subliminali neutri versus emotivi possa influenzare in qualche modo le risposte degli esaminati. Nello specifico, abbiamo reclutato un campione non clinico di 182 volontari adulti e abbiamo fornito loro il Difficulties in Emotion Regulation Questionnaire (DERS) e la Trait Meta-Mood Scale (TMMS). Successivamente, abbiamo somministrato loro il test di Rorschach utilizzando la seguente procedura sperimentale: ogni tavola Rorschach è stata presentata due volte sullo schermo di un computer, una volta in una condizione di priming subliminale neutro e una volta in una condizione di priming subliminale emotivo. Nella condizione di priming subliminale neutro, lo stimolo target del *backward masking* era una faccia neutra; nella condizione di priming subliminale emotivo, stimolo target del *backward masking* era una faccia arrabbiata. In entrambe le condizioni, lo stimolo target è rimasto sullo schermo per 10 m/s, quindi poteva essere processato solo a livello non consapevole. Le risposte dei partecipanti nelle condizioni di priming subliminale neutro versus priming subliminale emotivo sono state quindi esaminate e confrontate utilizzando il Rorschach Performance Assessment System (R-PAS). Inoltre, abbiamo anche voluto verificare l'ipotesi che gli individui con ridotte capacità di regolazione emotiva possano essere più suscettibili a piccole fluttuazioni emotive e quindi più influenzati dal priming subliminale. Abbiamo quindi testato una serie di ANCOVA con il priming (neutro versus emotivo) come fattore within-subject, i punteggi totali DERS e TMMS come covariate e ciascuno dei punteggi R-PAS di Pagina 1 e Pagina 2 come variabili dipendenti. I risultati hanno mostrato che i punteggi R-PAS ottenuti nelle condizioni di priming neutro ed emotivo erano notevolmente simili, indipendentemente dalla regolazione emotiva e dal livello di intelligenza emotiva dei partecipanti. Complessivamente, questi risultati suggeriscono che è improbabile che il priming subliminale influisca sul processo di risposta di Rorschach, sebbene siano necessari altri stimoli e progetti di ricerca per raggiungere tale conclusione con certezza.

Résumé

Les effets de l'amorçage émotionnel sur les réponses au test de Rorschach ont été peu étudiés dans la littérature. En particulier, aucune étude à ce jour n'a examiné si l'amorçage subliminal peut avoir un impact sur les processus de réponse de Rorschach. Pour combler cette lacune dans la littérature, nous avons utilisé un paradigme de masquage en arrière et testé si la présentation des taches de Rorschach après des stimuli subliminaux neutres ou émotionnels pouvait d'une manière ou d'une autre influencer les réponses des répondants. Plus précisément, nous avons recruté un échantillon non clinique de 182 volontaires adultes et leur avons fourni le questionnaire sur les Difficulties in Emotion Regulation Questionnaire (DERS) et l'échelle Trait Meta-Mood Scale (TMMS). Ensuite, nous leur avons administré le test de Rorschach en utilisant la procédure expérimentale suivante : Chaque tableau de Rorschach a été présenté deux fois sur un écran d'ordinateur, une fois dans une condition d'amorçage subliminal neutre et une fois dans une condition d'amorçage subliminal émotionnel. Dans la condition d'amorçage subliminal neutre, le stimulus cible du masquage arrière était un visage neutre; dans l'état d'amorçage subliminal émotionnel, le stimulus cible du masquage vers l'arrière était un visage en colère. Dans les deux conditions, le stimulus cible est resté sur l'écran pendant 10 m / s, il ne pouvait donc être traité qu'au niveau inconscient. Les réponses des participants dans les conditions d'amorçage subliminal neutre par rapport à l'amorçage subliminal émotionnel ont ensuite été examinées et comparées à l'aide du Rorschach Performance Assessment System (R-PAS). De plus, nous avons également voulu tester l'hypothèse selon laquelle les individus ayant une capacité de régulation émotionnelle réduite pourraient être plus sensibles aux petites fluctuations émotionnelles et donc plus influencés par l'amorçage subliminal. Nous avons ensuite testé une série d'ANCOVA avec l'amorçage (neutre versus émotionnel) comme facteur intra-sujet, les scores totaux DERS et TMMS comme covariables, et chacun des scores R-PAS comme variables dépendantes. Les résultats ont montré que les scores R-PAS obtenus dans les conditions d'amorçage neutre et émotionnel étaient remarquablement similaires, quel que soit le niveau de régulation émotionnelle et d'intelligence émotionnelle des participants. Dans l'ensemble, ces résultats suggèrent qu'il est peu probable que l'amorçage subliminal affecte le processus de réponse de Rorschach, bien que d'autres stimuli et projets de recherche soient nécessaires pour parvenir à cette conclusion avec certitude.

Resumen

Los efectos del priming emocional sobre las respuestas del test de Rorschach han sido poco estudiados en la literatura. En particular, ningún estudio hasta la fecha ha examinado si el subliminal priming puede tener un impacto en los procesos de respuesta de Rorschach. Para llenar este vacío en la literatura, utilizamos un paradigma de *backward masking* y probamos si presentar las manchas de Rorschach después de estímulos subliminales neutrales versus emocionales podría influir de alguna manera en las respuestas de los encuestados. Específicamente, reclutamos una muestra no clínica de 182 voluntarios adultos y les proporcionamos el Difficulties in Emotion Regulation Questionnaire (DERS) y la Trait Meta-Mood Scale (TMMS). A continuación, les administramos la prueba de Rorschach usando el siguiente procedimiento experimental: cada tablero de Rorschach se presentó dos veces en una pantalla de computadora, una vez en una condición de subliminal priming neutral y otra en una condición de subliminal priming emocional. En la condición de subliminal priming neutral, el estímulo objetivo del *backward masking* era una cara neutral; en la condición de subliminal priming emocional, el estímulo objetivo del *backward masking* era un rostro enojado. En ambas condiciones, el estímulo objetivo permaneció en la pantalla durante 10 m/s, por lo que solo pudo procesarse a nivel inconsciente. Las respuestas de los participantes en las condiciones de subliminal priming neutral versus subliminal priming emocional fueron luego examinadas y comparadas utilizando el Rorschach Performance Assessment System (R-PAS). Además, también queríamos probar la hipótesis de que las personas con capacidad de regulación emocional reducida pueden ser más susceptibles a pequeñas fluctuaciones emocionales y, por lo tanto, más influenciadas por el subliminal priming. Luego probamos una serie de ANCOVA con subliminal priming (neutral versus emocional) como factor dentro del sujeto, las puntuaciones totales de DERS y TMMS como covariables, y cada una de las puntuaciones R-PAS de la página 1 y la página 2 como variables dependientes. Los resultados mostraron que las puntuaciones R-PAS obtenidas en las condiciones de priming neutral y emocional fueron notablemente similares, independientemente del nivel de regulación emocional y de inteligencia emocional de los participantes. En general, estos hallazgos sugieren que es poco probable que el subliminal priming afecte el proceso de respuesta de Rorschach, aunque se necesitan otros estímulos y proyectos de investigación para llegar a esta conclusión con certeza.

要約

感情プライミングがロールシャッハの反応に及ぼす影響については、これまであまり研究されてこなかった。特に、サブリミナル・プライミングがロールシャッハの反応過程に影響を与えるかどうかを検討した研究はこれまでされてこなかった。そこで、われわれは、後方マスキング・パラダイムを用いて、中性的なサブリミナル・プライミングと感情サブリミナル・プライミングの後に、ロールシャッハのインクブロット・デザインを見せることで、異なるタイプの反応が誘発されるかどうかを検証した。具体的には、182名の非臨床群の成人ボランティアを集め、DERS(Difficulties in Emotion Regulation questionnaire)とTMMS（Trait Meta-Mood Scale）を渡し、記入してもらった。次に、以下の手順でロールシャッハテストを実施した。各ロールシャッハカードは、コンピュータ画面上に、中性プライミング条件下と感情プライミング条件下の2回提示された。中性サブリミナル条件では、後方マスキングの標的はニュートラルな顔であり、感情プライミング条件では、後方マスキングの標的は怒り顔であった。両条件とも、標的刺激は画面上に0.01秒間提示され、無意識的なレベルでのみ処理可能であった。そして、中性プライミング条件または感情プライミング条件における参加者の反応を、R-PASを用いて採点し、比較した。さらに、感情調節機能が低下している人は、小さな感情の変動に敏感であるため、サブリミナル・プライミングの影響を受けやすいのではないか、という仮説も検証したいと考えた。そこで、プライミング（中性対感情）を被験者内因子、DERSとTMMSの合計得点を共変量、1ページ目と2ページ目のR-PASのサマリースコアのそれぞれを従属変数として、一連の共分散分析を行った。その結果、中性プライミング条件と感情プライミング条件で得られたロールシャッハスコアは、参加者の感情調整や情緒的な知的のレベルに関わらず、驚くほど似ていることが示された。これらの結果をまとめると、サブリミナル・プライミングがロールシャッハの反応過程に影響を与える可能性は低いと考えられるが、そのような結論に達するには、他の刺激や研究デザインが必要である。

Original Article

The Specific Uses of the Rorschach in Clinical Practice

Preliminary Results From an International Survey

Joni L. Mihura[1], Callie E. Jowers[2], Nicolae Dumitrascu[3], Alicia W. Villanueva van den Hurk[4], and Philip J. Keddy[5,6]

[1]Department of Psychology, University of Toledo, OH, USA
[2]Department of Psychology, University of Detroit Mercy, MI, USA
[3]Albert & Jessie Danielsen Institute, Boston University, MA, USA
[4]Department of Psychology, University of Dayton, OH, USA
[5]Independent Practice, Oakland, CA, USA
[6]Wright Institute, Berkeley, CA, USA

Abstract: Our study addresses the question, "In what settings, with what age groups, and for what purposes is the Rorschach used internationally?" We present preliminary results from 342 Rorschach users representing 36 different countries from a survey created as part of the US contribution to a larger international project on teaching and using the Rorschach in different countries. The survey was distributed to R-PAS account holders with a request to forward to non-R-PAS users. Of the respondents, 80% used R-PAS, 35% used the CS, and 17% used both. Overall, 91% used the Rorschach with adults, and 43% and 69% with children and adolescents, respectively. The most common setting was private practice (63%). The most common reason for using the Rorschach was differential diagnosis (65%), with psychosis (58%) and personality disorders (56%) as the main diagnoses. US respondents were more likely to use the Rorschach to assess for psychosis (65% vs. 48%), especially emerging psychosis in adolescents (46% vs. 25%). We discuss the strong meta-analytic support for using the Rorschach to assess psychosis, a use supported by even the test's staunchest critics. We close by discussing study limitations and future directions, such as translating the survey to different languages and implementing a wider distribution.

Keywords: clinical practice, Rorschach, psychological assessment, psychosis

Since the first edition of Rorschach's *Psychodiagnostics* in 1921 (Rorschach, 1921/2021), his inkblot method widely spread across the globe. However, little is currently known about the specific purposes for which it is used in practice and for what age groups clinicians find it most helpful. These questions grew out of a project by a United States Task Force for the International Society of the Rorschach and Projective Techniques (ISR) for the centennial celebration of the Rorschach, scheduled for July 2022, to learn more about the history of how it came to various countries and where it was initially taught. For our part of this ISR project, we were only asked to report this information for the United States. We included other countries and questions about the use of the Rorschach in clinical practice due to our own interests in learning this additional information. Therefore, we created a survey to assess the settings, age groups, and purposes for which the Rorschach test is used internationally (e.g., differential diagnosis, assessing for psychosis or personality disorders). We were especially interested in the question, "When someone chooses to use the Rorschach, why or for what purposes is it is used?"

We located one published US survey, conducted in 2009, that included questions about the purposes for psychological assessment more broadly but not for individual tests specifically (Wright et al., 2017). The most common purpose for conducting a psychological assessment was to assist in making diagnostic decisions (85%). About half the respondents also reported using psychological assessment to address treatment impasses (47%), for forensic or psycholegal purposes (46%), and as a therapeutic intervention (40%; e.g., collaborative/therapeutic assessment (C/TA)).

In what follows, we report survey results on use of the Rorschach in clinical practice internationally, including the purposes, settings, and age groups for which it is used. Due to the large proportion of respondents from the United States, we also will evaluate whether the results differ between the United States and other countries.

Method

Survey Development and Implementation

This survey was initially developed as part of a larger project led by Emiliano Muzio (President of The Finnish Rorschach Association) in preparation for the International Society of the Rorschach and Projective Methods (ISR) centennial celebration of the birth of Hermann Rorschach's original publication of his inkblot test in 1921 and his death in 1922. Presidents of Rorschach societies in each country in the ISR were asked to respond to the following questions to trace the routes that the Rorschach spread across the world and where it is taught today (called the "MAP project"): When did the Rorschach come to your country?; Who brought it to your country?; What institutions taught and currently teach the Rorschach in your country? Because no Rorschach-specific US society exists, the President of the Society for Personality Assessment (SPA) gathered a US-based task force of SPA members (the authors of this article) to assist in the various ISR country projects for the United States. SPA was originally incorporated as the Rorschach Institute, Inc. in 1938, and the Society broadened its scope and changed its name to the Society for Personality Assessment in 1971. At this writing, in contrast to other countries in the ISR, no US-based Rorschach-specific professional society exists.

This SPA ISR Task Force also expanded the survey questions to obtain other information about how the Rorschach was used in clinical practice. Because R-PAS account holders are from a variety of countries, we also extended the focus beyond the United States to all account holders and any Rorschach user to which an account holder forwarded the survey. We know of no other country that conducted a formal survey like this. This is the initial publication of the survey results – specifically, for what settings, for which age groups, and for what purposes or referral questions is the Rorschach used internationally?

We created and administered the survey in PsychData.com. The survey was beta tested by 10 people from five different countries: United States, Italy, Norway, Spain, and Romania. The survey was distributed to Rorschach Performance Assessment System (R-PAS; Meyer et al., 2011) account holders, once in September 2021 and a second time in December 2021. We were interested in the use of any Rorschach system, not only R-PAS – in particular, the Comprehensive System (CS; Exner, 2003). However, we did not have access to such a distribution list. Therefore, the survey instructed respondents, "If you have colleagues who use a different Rorschach system, we would be grateful if you could forward this to them." The data we report in this article address the following questions: the respondents' country, which Rorschach system they use, in what settings they use the Rorschach, with what age groups, and the main purposes or referral questions for which the Rorschach is used. We provided multiple response options for these questions as well as the opportunity for the respondent to add their own category (an "Other" textbox). For all sections, respondents could choose as many options as they wished. We also analyzed the differences between the United States and other countries regarding our main research question: the response options for these questions are reported in the subsequent tables of results (a copy of the survey is available from the corresponding author). Of note, we offered "acute" and "long-term" inpatient response options, and some respondents added comments in the "Other" section, adding "residential treatment setting." Therefore, we combined across these categories to a general "inpatient/residential treatment" setting. Due to the number of statistical comparisons, we used an alpha level of $p < .01$ for statistical significance.

Results

Participants

Complete responses were received from 342 respondents. The median completion time was 3 min 29 s. Respondents were from the 36 countries shown in Table 1, which is organized by continent with the percentage of respondents per continent

Table 1. Countries represented in the survey

Continent/country	N	%
North America	209	61.1
Bermuda	1	0.3
Canada	8	2.3
Costa Rica	2	0.6
Mexico	1	0.3
Puerto Rico	2	0.6
United States	195	57.0
Europe	83	24.3
Belgium	5	1.5
Croatia	1	0.3
Denmark	2	0.6
Finland	10	2.9
France	1	0.3
Ireland	2	0.6
Italy	29	8.5
Netherlands	10	2.9
Norway	3	0.9
Portugal	1	0.3
Romania	2	0.6
Serbia	1	0.3
Slovenia	12	3.5
Sweden	3	0.9
Switzerland	1	0.3
United Kingdom	1	0.3
Asia	22	6.4
India	1	0.3
Indonesia	1	0.3
Iran	2	0.6
Israel	15	4.4
Philippines	2	0.6
United Arab Emirates	1	0.3
South America	20	5.8
Argentina	3	0.9
Brazil	14	4.1
Peru	3	0.9

(Continued on next page)

Table 1. (Continued)

Continent/country	N	%
Africa	6	1.8
Algeria	1	0.3
Rwanda	2	0.6
South Africa	3	0.9
Australia	2	0.6

Note. Total N = 342.

listed in descending order: North America (61.1%), Europe (24.3%), Asia (6.4%), South America (5.8%), Africa (1.8%), and Australia (0.6%). The five countries with the largest proportion of responses were, in descending order: United States (57.0%), Italy (8.5%), Israel (4.4%), Brazil (4.1%), and Slovenia (3.5%). Due to the large proportion of US responses, we also decided to run analyses to see whether results differed between the United States and other countries.

As shown in Table 2, 80.1% of respondents used R-PAS, 35.1% used the CS; 17.3% of these respondents reported using both the CS and R-PAS (e.g., supervising at a setting that uses one system while using the other in their own practice); and 2.0% used a different system (e.g., Klopfer, Passi Tognazzo). Most respondents were licensed psychologists versus a trainee (92.1%).

Settings and Age Groups

Table 3 reports the types of settings in which respondents who used the Rorschach in clinical practice worked. The most common setting was private practice (62.9%). The next most common settings or situations were, in descending order: forensic use (criminal or civil, 35.7%), outpatient clinic (30.7%), training setting (26.0%), inpatient or residential treatment center (20.5%), school psychology setting (7.6%), and university counseling center (4.7%). Two settings differed between the United States and other countries at the $p < .01$ level: Fewer US respondents reported using the Rorschach in forensic psychiatric hospitals and university counseling centers compared to non-US respondents. Although not specifically asked, in the Other section, many respondents clarified that their civil forensic use of the Rorschach was for child custody or parental evaluation purposes. As shown in Table 4, the Rorschach was used with the following age groups: children (43.0%), adolescents (69.3%), adults (90.6%) and, as a subset of adults, older adults (17.3%). Compared to non-US respondents, significantly more US respondents reported using the Rorschach with children ($r = .19$, $p = .0003$) and adolescents ($r = .19$, $p = .0004$).

Table 2. The Rorschach Performance Assessment System (R-PAS), Comprehensive System (CS), or other Rorschach systems

System	N	%
R-PAS	274	80.1%
CS	120	35.1%
Both	59	17.3%
Other	7	2.0%

Note. Total *N* = 342.

Table 3. Types of settings in which the Rorschach is used

Setting or situation	N	%	US (n = 195) %	Non-US (n = 147) %	US vs. Non-US r	US vs. Non-US p
Private practice	215	62.9	65.6	59.2	.07	.22
Forensic (any)	122	35.7	33.3	38.8	−.06	.30
Outpatient clinic	105	30.7	25.6	37.4	−.13	.02
Any training context	89	26.0	24.6	27.9	−.04	.50
Graduate training program	74	21.6	20.0	23.8	−.05	.40
Graduate externship	18	5.3	6.2	4.1	.05	.40
Other training	13	3.8	4.6	2.7	.05	.37
Inpatient/residential	70	20.5	16.4	25.9	−.12	.03
Acute inpatient hospital	40	11.7	8.7	15.6	−.11	.05
Long-term psychiatric hospital	31	9.1	7.2	11.6	−.08	.16
Forensic psychiatric hospital	18	5.3	2.6	8.8	−.14	.01*
School psychology	26	7.6	7.7	7.5	.00	.94
University counseling center	16	4.7	1.5	8.8	−.17	.01*
Other (e.g., FAA evaluations)	18	5.3	5.7	4.8		

Note. Total *N* = 342. *p < .01; **p < .001.

Purposes/Referral Questions for Which the Rorschach Is Used

As shown in Table 5, the most common purposes for which the Rorschach was used was for differential diagnosis (65.2%), which did not differ between US and non-US respondents. The second most frequent purpose for using the Rorschach was to assess for psychosis (57.6%): 44.7% assessing psychosis in adults and 36.8% detecting emerging psychosis in adolescents. US respondents

Table 4. Age groups for which the Rorschach is used

Age group	N	%	US (n = 195) %	Non-US (n = 147) %	US vs. Non-US r	p
Adults	310	90.6	89.2	92.5	−.06	.30
Older adults	59	17.3	20.5	12.9	.10	.07
Adolescents	237	69.3	76.9	59.2	.19	.01**
Children	147	43.0	51.3	32.0	.19	.01**

Note. Total N = 342. *p < .01; **p < .001.

Table 5. Purposes or referral questions for which the Rorschach is used in practice

Reason or referral question	N	%	US (n = 195) %	Non-US (n = 147) %	US vs. Non-US r	p
Differential diagnosis	223	65.2	67.7	61.9	.06	.27
Psychosis assessment (any)	197	57.6	65.1	47.6	.18	.01*
Adults	153	44.7	50.8	36.7	.14	.01*
Adolescents: early detection	126	36.8	45.6	25.2	.21	.01**
Complicated cases	195	57.0	63.6	48.3	.15	.01*
Personality disorders	191	55.8	50.3	63.3	−.13	.02
Regular assessment battery	176	51.7	52.8	50.3	.02	.65
Outpatient	148	43.3	46.4	39.5	.07	.20
Inpatient	55	16.1	10.8	23.1	−.17	.01*
Collaborative/therapeutic assessment	154	45.6	40.4	52.4	−.12	.03
Trauma	139	40.6	43.6	36.7	.07	.20
Therapy impasse	136	39.8	39.5	40.1	−.01	.90
Any forensic use	122	35.7	33.3	38.8	−.06	.30
Criminal forensic (any)	71	20.8	22.1	19.0	.04	.50
Violence risk assessment	57	16.7	16.4	17.0	−.01	.88
Forensic psychiatric hospital	18	5.3	2.6	8.8	−.14	.01*
Civil forensic outpatient	83	24.3	22.6	26.5	−.05	.40
Suicide risk assessment	95	27.8	25.1	31.3	−.07	.21
Neuropsychological	70	20.5	25.6	13.6	.15	.01*
Educational problems	42	12.3	12.8	11.6	.02	.73
Physical symptoms or pain	27	7.9	5.1	11.6	−.12	.03
Medication	25	7.3	9.7	4.1	.11	.05
Other	23	6.7	7.7	5.4		

Note. Total N = 342. *p < .01; **p < .001.

were significantly more likely to use the Rorschach to assess for psychosis, especially for detecting emerging psychosis in adolescents – the largest US versus non-US effect size difference across all purposes for using the test ($r = 0.21$, $p = .00009$). Because US respondents also reported using the Rorschach more frequently with adolescents, in general, than respondents from other countries, we also conducted analyses limiting the sample to respondents who used the Rorschach with adolescents. In this context, US respondents were still significantly more likely to use the Rorschach to assess for emerging psychosis in adolescents (57.3%) compared to other countries (39.1%; $r = 0.18$, $p = 0.0066$). There were not enough data to conduct per-country analyses, but when aggregating the data across continents with at least 10 respondents who worked with adolescents, the percentage using the Rorschach to assess for emerging psychosis in adolescents was North America (57.2%, $n = 159$), Europe (40%, $n = 45$), Asia (33.3%, $n = 19$), and South America (27.3%, $n = 11$).

The third most frequent reason for using the Rorschach in clinical practice was for what we called "complicated cases" (57.0%), with US respondents reporting this usage more frequently than non-US respondents ($r = 0.15$, $p = .0046$). Other reasons reported by one third or more of the sample were to assess for personality disorders (55.8%), as part of a regular battery (51.7%), in a collaborative/therapeutic assessment (45.6%), in a trauma assessment (40.6%), in cases of therapeutic impasse (39.8), and for forensic purposes (35.7%). US and non-US respondents did not differ across these reasons. However, non-US respondents reported using the Rorschach as part of a regular assessment battery in inpatient settings more often than US respondents and using the Rorschach as part of a neuropsychological assessment less often than US respondents. When limiting the analyses to only respondents who work in and use the Rorschach in an inpatient setting (53.2%), there were no US/non-US differences in whether the Rorschach was included in a regular assessment battery in that setting (around 50%).

We were also curious as to the most common reasons for using the Rorschach when it is not already part of a regular assessment battery. The most common reasons ($\geq 50\%$), in descending order, were: differential diagnosis (60%), to assess for psychosis (53.3%), for complicated cases (52.1%), and to assess for personality disorders (50%). As with the full sample, US respondents were significantly more likely than non-US respondents to include the Rorschach in an assessment battery specifically to assess for psychosis (66.3% vs. 37.0%; $r = 0.29$, $p = .00014$). This was especially true when assessing for emerging psychosis in adolescents (47.8% vs. 17.8%; $r = 0.31$, $p = .000041$) compared to assessing for psychosis in adults (50% vs. 31.5%; $r = 0.19$, $p = .0166$), although with a small effect difference (Cohen's $q = 0.137$; Cohen, 1988).

Discussion

We obtained results from 36 countries on the uses of the Rorschach in clinical practice using an English-language survey sent to R-PAS account holders with instructions to forward to people who use other Rorschach systems. This is a preliminary survey that we intend to eventually translate to other languages and distribute through other outlets. Most respondents reported using R-PAS (80%), about a third used the CS (35%), and 17% of these respondents reported using both the CS and R-PAS; 2% reported using another Rorschach system.

The great majority of respondents reported using the Rorschach with adults (91%). The Rorschach was also used with adolescents (69%) and children (43%). US respondents were significantly more likely to use the Rorschach with children and adolescents compared to non-US respondents. Regarding the settings in which people who use the Rorschach employ its use, the most common setting was private practice (63%). Other settings and situations were for forensic purposes (36%), in outpatient clinics (31%), training contexts (26%), inpatient or residential treatment centers (21%), and under 10% for school psychology settings, university counseling centers, and others. The only two setting differences between US and non-US respondents were a smaller proportion of US respondents using the Rorschach in a forensic psychiatric hospital and in a university counseling center. It is important to note that these results do not indicate the proportion of psychologists in these settings who use the Rorschach but the proportion of Rorschach-using psychologists who use the Rorschach in these settings. For example, the results do not indicate the proportion of psychologists in private practice who use the Rorschach but, of psychologists who use the Rorschach, the proportion who use it in a private practice setting.

The most common purposes (> 50%) for which the Rorschach was used were, in descending order: for differential diagnosis, to assess for psychosis, for complicated cases, to assess for personality disorders, and as part of a regularly conducted assessment battery. Limiting the results to non-US respondents, using the Rorschach in a collaborative/therapeutic assessment enters into the most common purposes as defined by more than 50% of respondents. US respondents were less likely to use the Rorschach in a regular inpatient assessment battery. However, this difference was largely due to US respondents being less likely to report using the Rorschach in an inpatient setting to begin with. When we limited analyses to only respondents who used the Rorschach in an inpatient setting, the United States and other countries were equivalent in using the Rorschach in a regularly conducted assessment battery.

Using the Rorschach for Assessing Psychosis

We were pleased to see the frequent usage of using the Rorschach to assess for psychosis, because using the Rorschach for this purpose is *strongly* supported by research, including two systematic reviews and meta-analyses (Jørgensen et al., 2000, 2001; Mihura et al., 2013). The most recent and comprehensive meta-analyses found that the Rorschach psychosis index differentiated psychotic patients from nonpatients (d = 2.08, 95% CI [1.50, 2.87]) and from nonpsychotic patients (d = 1.07, 95% CI [0.75, 1.39]) with large effects (converted from the r values in Table 4 in Mihura et al., 2013). Research published after the Mihura et al. meta-analyses were conducted found that the R-PAS psychosis index (TP-Comp) shows an even stronger effect than the previous version (PTI in the CS) in differentiating psychotic from nonpsychotic patients (ds = 2.16 vs. 1.07) with statistically significant incremental validity ($\Delta\chi^2$ = 20.57, p < .001; Dzamonja-Ignjatovic et al., 2013) and significantly higher associations with measures of psychosis and psychopathology severity (M rs = .55 > .36, p = .012; from Tables 3 and 4; Su et al., 2015). Several contemporary resources exist for using the Rorschach to assess psychotic phenomena (Kleiger, 2017; Kleiger & Mihura, 2021; Meyer & Mihura, 2021).

Due to the potential deleterious effects of psychosis, the importance of early identification, and the strong support of the Rorschach for assessing psychosis – especially the disorganized thinking as seen in schizophrenia (Biagiarelli et al., 2015; Eblin et al., 2018; Kleiger & Mihura, 2021; Mihura et al., 2021; Mihura & Meyer, 2021) – it is imperative that mental health professionals overcome negative misperceptions of the Rorschach. Schizophrenia-spectrum disorders before age 18 can be more chronic, debilitating, and likely to be accompanied by other disorders; therefore, early identification is important (Biederman et al., 2004; Stentebjerg-Olesen et al., 2016). R-PAS and CS test variables designed to assess psychotic symptoms – visual misperceptions (FQ-%/X-%), disordered thinking (WSumCog/WSum6), and the related composite index (TP-Comp/PTI) – are the only psychosis measures used in clinical practice (Wright et al., 2017) that have published meta-analytic support for their validity (Mihura et al., 2013). In fact, results from unpublished meta-analyses raise flags about using the traditional MMPI/MMPI-2 Schizophrenia scale (Scale 8) to detect psychosis in a clinical setting with an effect magnitude of d = 0.00; a scale (Bizarre Mentation) more specifically targeting the symptoms of psychosis fared slightly better (d = .32; Mihura et al., 2016). When the literature review was conducted for these MMPI meta-analyses, there were an insufficient number of relevant studies using the newer versions of the test (MMPI-2-RF, MMPI-3). Studies also support the incremental validity of the Rorschach in detecting psychosis over these MMPI scales (Dao et al., 2008; Meyer, 2000; Ritsher, 2004).

Finally, people who criticize the Rorschach should be made aware of this research as well as the fact that even the Rorschach's staunchest critics have repeatedly supported using the Rorschach for assessing psychotic symptoms. For example, "There is abundant evidence that two kinds of Rorschach scores are related to psychotic disorders" (Wood et al., 2003). "Even psychologists who are critical of the test generally agree that some scores from various Rorschach systems can be helpful for detecting thought disorder [and] diagnosing mental disorders characterized by thought disorder" (Garb et al., 2005). Therefore, one negative consequence of publicized criticisms of the Rorschach (e.g., Garb, 1999; Wood et al., 1996, 2003) is the inaccurate conclusion that the Rorschach itself is invalid, which robs patients with emerging psychosis of the test that is taught and used in clinical practice (Mihura et al., 2017; Wright et al., 2017) with the best empirical support for assessing psychosis. Boyette and Noordhof (2021) – two previous skeptics of the Rorschach – state in their commentary on Kleiger and Mihura's (2021) article "Developments in the Rorschach Assessment of Disordered Thinking and Communication" that: "The Rorschach is valid and reliable for the assessment of disordered thinking and communication . . . and should no longer be harshly judged on criteria that are not typically met by alternatives" (p. 286).

Limitations and Future Directions

A key limitation to our study was conducting an international survey using an English-language survey. The impetus of our study was the US projects for the ISR centennial celebration and was, thus, initially focused on the Rorschach in the United States. We plan to follow up with translations of the survey to other languages to expand the scope and generalizability of our survey findings. In the meantime, our findings are generalizable to the global aggregate of the countries represented in the survey, not all the countries in which the Rorschach is used. The survey could also benefit from input from Rorschach users from countries not represented by our beta testers who reviewed our survey content, especially to identify additional response options and clarify existing ones. Another study limitation was relying solely on the R-PAS distribution list, although we instructed respondents to forward the survey to non-R-PAS users, the great majority of whom used the CS. A future survey could potentially use ISR and SPA distribution lists, for example.

Summary and Conclusion

We report the results of the first survey (of which we are aware) regarding the specific uses of the Rorschach in clinical practice. Our results show that the test is used in many different settings. The most common reason for using the Rorschach was for differential diagnosis, with psychosis as the main diagnostic differential. Future surveys should investigate why non-US countries were significantly less likely to use the Rorschach to assess for emerging psychosis in adolescents, especially due to the potential deleterious nature of the disorder and the strong empirical support for using the Rorschach to assess psychotic symptoms. Future surveys should also be distributed across a range of outlets and translated to different languages to extend the scope.

References

Biagiarelli, M., Roma, P., Comparelli, A., Andraos, M. P., Di Pomponio, I., Corigliano, V., Curto, M., Masters, G. A., & Ferracuti, S. (2015). Relationship between the Rorschach Perceptual Thinking Index (PTI) and the Positive and Negative Syndrome Scale (PANSS) in psychotic patients: A validity study. *Psychiatry Research, 225*(3), 315–321. https://doi.org/10.1016/j.psychres.2014.12.018

Biederman, J., Petty, C., Faraone, S. V., & Seidman, L. (2004). Phenomenology of childhood psychosis: Findings from a large sample of psychiatrically referred youth. *Journal of Nervous and Mental Disease, 192*(9), 607–614. https://doi.org/10.1097/01.nmd.0000138228.59938.c3

Boyette, L.-L., & Noordhof, A. (2021). A commentary on "Developments in the Rorschach assessment of disordered thinking and communication" (Kleiger & Mihura, 2021). *Rorschachiana, 42*(2), 281–288. https://doi.org/10.1027/1192-5604/a000145

Cohen, J. (1988). *Statistical power analysis for the behavioral sciences* (2nd ed.). Routledge.

Dao, T. K., Prevatt, F., & Horne, H. L. (2008). Differentiating psychotic patients from nonpsychotic patients with the MMPI-2 and Rorschach. *Journal of Personality Assessment, 90*(1), 93–101. https://doi.org/10.1080/00223890701693819

Dzamonja-Ignjatovic, T., Smith, B. L., Jocic, D. D., & Milanovic, M. (2013). A comparison of new and revised Rorschach measures of schizophrenic functioning in a Serbian clinical sample. *Journal of Personality Assessment, 95*(5), 471–478. https://doi.org/10.1080/00223891.2013.810153

Eblin, J. J., Meyer, G. J., Mihura, J. L., Viglione, D. J., & O'Gorman, E. T. (2018). Development and preliminary validation of a brief behavioral measure of psychotic propensity. *Psychiatry Research, 268*, 340–347. https://doi.org/10.1016/j.psychres.2018.08.006

Exner, J. E. (2003). *The Rorschach: A comprehensive system* (4th ed). John Wiley & Sons.

Garb, H. N. (1999). Call for a moratorium on the use of the Rorschach Inkblot Test in clinical and forensic settings. *Assessment, 6*(4), 313–317. https://doi.org/10.1177/107319119900600402

Garb, H. N., Wood, J. M., Lilienfeld, S. O., & Nezworski, M. T. (2005). Roots of the Rorschach controversy. *Clinical Psychology Review, 25*(1), 97–118. https://doi.org/10.1016/j.cpr.2004.09.002

Jørgensen, K., Andersen, T. J., & Dam, H. (2000). The diagnostic efficiency of the Rorschach Depression Index and the Schizophrenia Index: A review. *Assessment, 7*(3), 259–280. https://doi.org/10.1177/107319110000700306

Jørgensen, K., Andersen, T. J., & Dam, H. (2001). The diagnostic efficiency of the Rorschach Depression Index and the Schizophrenia Index: A review [Erratum]. *Assessment, 8*(3), 355. https://doi.org/10.1177/107319110100800311

Kleiger, J. H. (2017). *Rorschach assessment of psychotic phenomena: Clinical, conceptual, and empirical developments*. Routledge/Taylor & Francis Group.

Kleiger, J. H., & Mihura, J. L. (2021). Developments in the Rorschach assessment of disordered thinking and communication. *Rorschachiana, 42*(2), 265–280. https://doi.org/10.1027/1192-5604/a000132

Meyer, G. J. (2000). On the science of Rorschach research. *Journal of Personality Assessment, 75*(1), 46–81. https://doi.org/10.1207/S15327752JPA7501_6

Meyer, G. J., & Mihura, J. L. (2021). Rorschach Performance Assessment System (R-PAS) for assessing disordered thought and perception. In I. B. Weiner & J. H. Kleiger (Eds.), *Psychological assessment of disordered thinking and perception* (pp. 151–168). American Psychological Association. https://doi.org/10.1037/0000245-010

Meyer, G. J., Viglione, D. J., Mihura, J. L., Erard, R. E., & Erdberg, P. (2011). *Rorschach Performance Assessment System: Administration, coding, interpretation, and technical manual*. Rorschach Performance Assessment System, LLC.

Mihura, J. L., Roy, M., Dumitrascu, N., & Meyer, G. J. (2016, March 12). *A meta-analytic review of the MMPI (all versions) ability to detect psychosis*. Paper presented at the Annual Meeting of the Society for Personality Assessment, Chicago, IL, USA.

Mihura, J. L., & Meyer, G. J. (2021). The Rorschach Performance Assessment System (R-PAS) in multimethod assessment. In J. L. Mihura (Ed.), *The Oxford Handbook of Personality and Psychopathology Assessment* (2nd ed.). Oxford University Press.

Mihura, J. L., Meyer, G. J., Dumitrascu, N., & Bombel, G. (2013). The validity of individual Rorschach variables: Systematic reviews and meta-analyses of the comprehensive system. *Psychological Bulletin, 139*(3), 548–605. https://doi.org/10.1037/a0029406

Mihura, J. L., Meyer, G. J., Viglione, D. J., Kletzka, N., Eblin, J. J., Boyette, L.-L., Kleiger, J. H., & Ales, F. (2021). *Validating a standardized measure of disorganized thinking using the Rorschach*. Manuscript in preparation.

Mihura, J. L., Roy, M., & Graceffo, R. A. (2017). Psychological assessment training in clinical psychology doctoral programs. *Journal of Personality Assessment, 99*(2), 153–164. https://doi.org/10.1080/00223891.2016.1201978

Ritsher, J. B. (2004). Association of Rorschach and MMPI psychosis indicators and schizophrenia spectrum diagnoses in a Russian clinical sample. *Journal of Personality Assessment, 83*(1), 46–63. https://doi.org/10.1207/s15327752jpa8301_05

Rorschach, H. (2021). *Hermann Rorschach's psychodiagnostics: Newly translated and annotated 100th anniversary edition* (P. J. Keddy, R. Signer, P. Erdberg, & A. Schneider-Stocking, Trans. & Eds.). Hogrefe Publishing. (Original work published 1921)

Stentebjerg-Olesen, M., Pagsberg, A. K., Fink-Jensen, A., Correll, C. U., & Jeppesen, P. (2016). Clinical characteristics and predictors of outcome of schizophrenia-spectrum psychosis in children and adolescents: A systematic review. *Journal of Child and Adolescent Psychopharmacology, 26*(5), 410–427. https://doi.org/10.1089/cap.2015.0097

Su, W.-S., Viglione, D. J., Green, E. E., Tam, W.-C. C., Su, J.-A., & Chang, Y.-T. (2015). Cultural and linguistic adaptability of the Rorschach Performance Assessment System as a measure of psychotic characteristics and severity of mental disturbance in Taiwan. *Psychological Assessment, 27*(4), 1273–1285. https://doi.org/10.1037/pas0000144

Wood, J. M., Nezworski, M. T., Lilienfeld, S. O., & Garb, H. N. (2003). *What's wrong with the Rorschach?: Science confronts the controversial inkblot test.* Jossey-Bass.

Wood, J. M., Nezworski, M. T., & Stejskal, W. J. (1996). The comprehensive system for the Rorschach: A critical examination. *Psychological Science, 7*(1), 3–10. https://doi.org/10.1111/j.1467-9280.1996.tb00658.x

Wright, C. V., Beattie, S. G., Galper, D. I., Church, A. S., Bufka, L. F., Brabender, V. M., & Smith, B. L. (2017). Assessment practices of professional psychologists: Results of a national survey. *Professional Psychology: Research and Practice, 48*(2), 73–78. https://doi.org/10.1037/pro0000086

History
Received December 12, 2021
Revision received January 24, 2022
Accepted January 30, 2022
Published online April 28, 2022

Conflict of Interest
The first author is a part owner of a company that publishes the Rorschach Performance Assessment System® (R-PAS®) test manual (Meyer et al., 2011) and associated products.

ORCID
Joni L. Mihura
 https://orcid.org/0000-0003-0627-9869
Callie E. Jowers
 https://orcid.org/0000-0003-1395-4025
Nicolae Dumitrascu
 https://orcid.org/0000-0003-0837-8983
Alicia W. Villanueva van den Hurk
 https://orcid.org/0000-0002-9026-3298
Philip J. Keddy
 https://orcid.org/0000-0003-1892-0043

Joni L. Mihura
Department of Psychology
University of Toledo
2801 W. Bancroft Dr., MS 948
Toledo, OH 43606
USA
joni.mihura@utoledo.edu

Summary

Our study addresses the question, "In what settings, with what age groups, and for what purposes is the Rorschach used internationally?" This is the first such study of which we are aware. The survey started as part of the US contribution to the 100th centennial celebration of the Rorschach by the International Society for the Rorschach and Projective Methods (ISR) planned for taking place in Geneva, Switzerland in 2022, and was limited to the English language and distributed to Rorschach Performance Assessment System (R-PAS; Meyer et al., 2011) account holders. We present survey results from 342 respondents, representing 36 different countries, who use the

Rorschach in clinical practice. Respondents were 80.1% R-PAS users and 35.1% Comprehensive System (CS; Exner, 2003) users (17.3% of these respondents reported using both the CS and R-PAS); 2.0% reported using other systems. About half were from the US (57%). Overall, 91% used the Rorschach with adults, and 43% and 69% with children and adolescents, respectively. The most common setting was private practice (63%). Other settings, in descending order of frequency, were forensic, outpatient clinics, training contexts, inpatient or residential treatment centers, school psychology settings, and university counseling centers. The most common reason for using the Rorschach was differential diagnosis (65%). Using the Rorschach to assess for psychosis, specifically, was next most frequent (58%) although several other uses were comparable (e.g., for complicated cases, part of a regularly conducted assessment battery, collaborative/therapeutic assessments, therapy impasses, forensic assessments). Compared to other countries, US respondents were more likely to use the Rorschach to assess for psychosis (65% vs. 48%), especially emerging psychosis in adolescents (46% vs. 25%), whereas using the Rorschach to assess personality disorders was essentially tied with differential diagnosis more broadly as the most common reasons in non-US countries (63% vs. 62%). We discuss the strong meta-analytic support for using the Rorschach to assess psychosis, a use supported by even the test's staunchest critics. We close by discussing limitations of the survey and future directions. In particular, a goal for the future is to translate the survey to different languages and implement a wider distribution.

Résumé

Notre étude aborde la question suivante : "Dans quels contextes, avec quels groupes d'âge et à quelles fins le Rorschach est-il utilisé au niveau international ?" Il s'agit de la première étude de ce type dont nous avons connaissance. L'enquête a été lancée dans le cadre de la contribution américaine à la célébration du 100e centenaire du Rorschach par la Société internationale pour le Rorschach et les méthodes projectives (ISR) prévue à Genève, en Suisse, en 2022, et a été limitée à la langue anglaise et distribuée aux détenteurs de comptes Rorschach Performance Assessment System (R-PAS; Meyer et al., 2011). Nous présentons les résultats de l'enquête auprès de 342 répondants, représentant 36 pays différents, qui utilisent le Rorschach dans la pratique clinique. Les répondants étaient 80,1% à utiliser le R-PAS et 35,1% à utiliser le Comprehensive System (CS; Exner, 2003) (17,3% de ces répondants ont déclaré utiliser à la fois le CS et le R-PAS); 2,0% ont déclaré utiliser d'autres systèmes. Environ la moitié des répondants étaient originaires des États-Unis (57%). Quatre-vingt-onze pour cent ont utilisé le Rorschach avec des adultes, et 43% et 69% avec des enfants et des adolescents, respectivement. Le cadre le plus courant était le cabinet privé (63%). Les autres milieux, par ordre décroissant de fréquence, étaient la médecine légale, les cliniques externes, les contextes de formation, les centres de traitement pour patients hospitalisés ou en résidence, les milieux de la psychologie scolaire et les centres de conseil universitaires. La raison la plus fréquente de l'utilisation du Rorschach était le diagnostic différentiel (65%). L'utilisation du Rorschach pour évaluer la psychose, spécifiquement, était ensuite la plus fréquente (58%) bien que plusieurs autres utilisations étaient comparables (par exemple, pour les cas compliqués, les troubles de la personnalité, et dans le cadre d'une batterie d'évaluation régulière). Comparé aux autres pays, les répondants américains étaient plus susceptibles d'utiliser le Rorschach pour évaluer la psychose (65% vs. 48%), en particulier la psychose émergente chez les adolescents (46% vs. 25%), tandis que l'utilisation du Rorschach pour évaluer les troubles de la personnalité était essentiellement à égalité avec le diagnostic différentiel plus largement comme les raisons les plus courantes dans les pays non-américains (63% & 62%). Nous discutons du fort soutien méta-analytique pour l'utilisation du Rorschach pour évaluer la psychose, une utilisation soutenue même par les plus farouches critiques du test. Nous terminons en discutant des limites de l'enquête et des orientations futures. En particulier, un objectif pour l'avenir est de traduire l'enquête dans différentes langues et de mettre en œuvre une distribution plus large.

Resumen

Nuestro estudio responde a la pregunta, "¿En qué entorno, con qué grupos de edades, y con qué propósito se usa el Rorschach internacionalmente?" Éste es el primer estudio de este tipo del que tenemos conocimiento. La encuesta empezó como parte de la contribución estadounidense a la celebración del 100 aniversario del Rorschach, organizado por la International Society for the Rorschach and Projective Methods (ISR), que tendrá lugar en Ginebra, Suiza en 2022, y fue limitada a la lengua inglesa y distribuida a titulares de cuentas del Rorschach Performance Assessment System (R-PAS; Meyer et al., 2011). Nosotros presentamos resultados de 342 encuestados, representando 36 países diferentes, los cuales usan el Rorschach en práctica clínica. Un 80.1% de los respondientes usaban R-PAS y un 35.1% usaban el Comprehensive System (CS; Exner, 2003) (17.3% de los cuales afirmaron usar tanto el CS como el R-PAS); el 2.0% afirmaron usar otros sistemas. Aproximadamente la mitad eran de Estados Unidos (57%). El noventa y uno por ciento usaban el Rorschach con adultos, y el 43% y el 69% con niños y adolescentes, respectivamente. El entorno más común fueron prácticas privadas (63%). Otros entornos, en orden descendente por frecuencia, fueron forenses, clínicas de consulta externa, contextos de formación, pacientes internos o centros de tratamiento residencial, entornos de psicología escolar, y centros de terapia en universidades. La razón más común para usar el Rorschach fue para hacer diagnósticos diferenciales (65%). La siguiente razón más frecuente para usar el Rorschach fue para evaluar específicamente psicosis (58%), aunque había varios otros usos con cifras similares (p. ej., para casos complicados, como parte de un conjunto de evaluaciones realizadas regularmente, evaluaciones colaborativas/terapéuticas, estancamiento en terapia, evaluaciones forenses). En comparación con otros países, los encuestados de Estados Unidos eran más propensos a usar el Rorschach para evaluar psicosis (65% vs. 48%), especialmente en adolescentes con psicosis emergente (46% vs. 25%), mientras que el uso del Rorschach para evaluar trastornos de personalidad estaba esencialmente vinculado con diagnósticos diferenciales más amplios que las razones más comunes en aquellos países diferentes a Estados Unidos (63% y 62%). Nosotros hablamos del fuerte respaldo meta-analítico para usar el Rorschach para evaluar psicosis, un uso que esté apoyado incluso por los críticos más firmes de este test. Nosotros finalizamos hablando de las limitaciones de la encuesta y de direcciones futuras. En particular, un objetivo para el futuro es traducir la encuesta a diferentes idiomas e implementar una distribución más amplia.

要約

本研究では、「国際的にロールシャッハはどのような場面で、どのような年齢層で、どのような目的で使用されているのか?」という問いに取り組んでいる。私たちが知る限り、このような研究はこれまでに見られない。この調査は、2022年にスイスのジュネーブで開催される国際ロールシャッハ及び投映法学会 (ISR) 100年記念大会のプロジェクトの中でアメリカの担当部分として開始され、英語に限定して、Rorschach Performance Assessment System(R-PAS; Meyerら, 2011) のアカウントを持つ者にアンケートが配布された。臨床でロールシャッハを使用している36カ国、342名の回答者からの結果を提示する。回答者の内訳は、R-PASユーザーが80.1%、包括システム (CS; Exner, 2003) が35.1% (このうち、17.3%がCSとR-PASの両方を使用していると回答) 、その他のシステムを使用していると回答したのは2.0%であった。また、約半数がアメリカからの回答であった (57%) 。ロールシャッハの対象者について、91%が成人、43%が子どもに、69%が青年に使用していると回答した。どこで使用しているかについ

て、最も多かったのが開業（63%）であった。その他、使用頻度の高い順に、法医学、外来クリニック、研修の場、入院または入所治療施設、スクールカウンセリング、大学の学生相談室であった。ロールシャッハを使用する目的で最も多かったのは、鑑別診断（65%）であった。次に多かったのは、精神病の評価に用いることであったが（58%）、他の用途はほぼ同程度の割合であった（例：複雑なケース、定期的に行うテストバッテリーの一部、協働的/治療的アセスメントのツールとして、治療の行き詰まり、法医学評価など）。他国と比較して、アメリカの回答者は、精神病の評価（65%対48%）、特に青年期発症の精神病（46%対25%）にロールシャッハを用いる傾向が強かった。一方、アメリカ以外の国では、ロールシャッハを使用してパーソナリティ障害を評価することが、より広範な鑑別診断とほぼ同じであった（63%対62%）。ロールシャッハを精神病の評価に使用することが、メタアナリシスによって強く支持され、このテストを最も厳しく批評する人たちからでさえも支持されていることについて報告する。最後に、本調査の限界と今後の方向性について述べる。特に今後の課題は、この調査をさまざまな言語に翻訳し、より広く調査することである。

Original Article

On Psychosis

An International Comparative Single Case Study
of the Nancy French, Lausanne, and American
Rorschach Approaches

Cécile Prudent[1], James H. Kleiger[2], Odile Husain[3],
and Claude De Tychey[4]

[1]Private Practice, Marseille, France
[2]Private Practice, Bethesda, MD, USA
[3]Private Practice, Montreal, QC, Canada
[4]Laboratory interpsy EA4432, University of Lorraine, Nancy, France

Abstract: This manuscript presents a single case study of a psychotically disturbed adult male (whom we call "Peter"), focusing on similarities and differences in Rorschach interpretation based on three different Rorschach approaches. Specific questions were raised as to whether the client suffered from a paranoid psychosis (paranoia) or paranoid schizophrenia. Three distinct models of psychopathology and Rorschach interpretation are initially presented. We then address Peter's psychotic symptoms, according to the Parisian approach (specifically the Nancy French subgroup), the Lausanne Rorschach approach, and the American Rorschach approach (Comprehensive System and R-PAS). Analysis shows many convergences between the three approaches on the client's nature of conflicts and links to reality, object relations, self-representation and anxiety, defense mechanisms, and disordered thinking, but interpretation of these variables differed somewhat despite agreement on a diagnosis within the psychotic spectrum. Concluding remarks discuss the divergences and point out the limitations of a case study method. Future research is suggested.

Keywords: Rorschach, psychoanalysis, psychosis, paranoia

With diversity among Rorschach methods, systems, models, and underlying theories, how much convergence in diagnostic understanding can occur among different clinicians who ascribe to distinct psychodiagnostic traditions? We addressed this question by comparing and contrasting multiple approaches to interpreting psychological testing material in the context of a clinical case presentation. We narrowed the focus by examining differential diagnostic issues related to psychosis and by exploring where the traditions, models, and theories from different culture-specific approaches diverged and where they coalesced in our efforts to gain diagnostic clarity.

Rorschachiana (2022), 43(1), 42–69
https://doi.org/10.1027/1192-5604/a000151

Clinicians from three relatively distinct psychodiagnostic cultures or traditions, the Nancy French, Lausanne, and American approaches, provide an overview of their methods and apply their systems, models, and theories to the interpretation of the Rorschach of a 37-year-old patient, called "Peter," who had previously been diagnosed within the psychotic spectrum (see Appendix for a brief anamnesis). Although the actual assessment of Peter included multiple methods, in this paper we place more emphasis on the Rorschach, which has long been shown to be a powerful method for assessing psychotic symptoms and structures (Holzman et al., 1986; Kleiger, 2017; Mihura et al., 2013).

Theoretical Background of Three Rorschach Approaches

Although there is diversity among the approaches, all three have a long tradition of teaching and advanced training in the Rorschach. Despite their differences, both the Nancy and Lausanne systems are homogeneous and rooted in a model of psychopathology and theoretical framework. By contrast, the American approach includes a looser, less well-articulated federation of Rorschach approaches which, over time, have become more centered on specific psychometric methodology, decoupled from theoretical interpretation. Despite the absence of a clearly defined American system, we summarize the approaches that can be more defined in the tradition of American psychodiagnosticians interested in studying psychosis.

Nancy French Approach Belonging to Parisian Approach

Theoretical and methodological diversity can be seen inside the three principal groups of the Parisian approach (University of Paris Descartes, University of Nancy Lorraine, and University of Lyon Lumière II). These three consortia share the same Rorschach coding methodology and base their projective interpretation on a theoretical psychoanalytic model but significant differences also exist between them. According to Jean Bergeret (1974), everyone has a personality structure, and each personality structure can express itself in a normal mode through a character corresponding to the structure, or in a pathological mode when the personality structure decompensates as a result of a traumatic event or history. However, each organizational mode on the intrapsychic level is defined by stable markers, such as dominant anxiety, specific defense mechanisms against anxiety, dominant object relations, specific libidinal organization level of the self, nature of conflict, and link with reality. When confronted with the failings of repression, the prevalent psychotic defense mechanisms are projection, denial of reality, splitting, and dissociation of the Ego. For Bergeret, these defense mechanisms are responsible for the phenomenon of depersonalization and personality dissociation and are involved in the genesis of thought disorders. On the clinical level (see anamnesis in Appendix), Peter, the case we are presenting, simultaneously poses the problem of differential diagnosis between schizophrenia and paranoia and the psychotic status of paranoia as a dissociated psychosis. For Bergeret, the schizophrenic structure occupies, in terms of the instinctual economy, a more regressive position (oral stage) than the paranoiac structure (first anal substage). There exists in the paranoiac structure a repressed homosexual desire that leads to projection and the feeling of persecution. The nature of conflicts, for both the schizophrenic and paranoiac structures, is a conflict between instincts and reality. The nature of fragmentation anxiety, dominant in all psychotic structures, is nonetheless different within each structure. In the schizophrenic structure, fragmentation anxiety results from the lack of unity with the body Ego, whereas in the paranoiac structure, fragmentation anxiety is sparked by fears of anal penetration. Schizophrenic structure has an object relation centered on fusion, whereas the paranoiac individual is able to establish an object relation with an object clearly differenciated but invested in a persecutory fashion.

Stable markers of Bergeret's model are illustrated by the Rorschach test. We added a section related to disordered thinking, which constitutes a central dimension for the Lausanne and American approaches.

The Lausanne Approach

The Lausanne approach was founded by a French-Swiss group which started developing a qualitative analysis of the Rorschach and the Thematic Apperception Test (TAT) in the late 1970s based on Bergeret's (1974) writings. In the 1980s, the exposure to Piagetian concepts (1966) further expanded the method. The Lausanne approach aimed at differentiating personality organizations as conceptualized by Bergeret. Currently, the method is referred to as "psychodynamic analysis of speech." The Lausanne members' objective was to analyze the greatest *quantity* of speech possible, hence the choice of a qualitative approach, which can take into consideration both frequent and rare signs (Barthes, 1980), as well as nonscorable parts of speech. Consequently, the method does not use a scoring system per se, but a grid with six columns (object relations, boundaries, self-representation, anxiety, defense mechanisms, thought disorders): Responses and other verbalizations are listed within the grid. The Lausanne approach promotes the use of the same grid for both Rorschach and TAT, thus enabling convergences to be established. The Lausanne approach integrates other theoretical models: Racamier's (1980) psychoanalytical understanding of schizophrenic thought, Piaget's considerations on representation, and Bohm's (1955/1985) concept of interpretive awareness, as well as traditional thought disorders observed on the Rorschach to understand these cognitive processes.

Comparison of the Nancy French with the Lausanne approach's interpretations will be even more interesting because the latter also uses Bergeret's theoretical model (contrary to the two other French groups of Paris Descartes and Lyon, who have a more processual approach of Rorschach data interpretation and other psychoanalytic references). However, the Lausanne approach has a more integrative approach, since it is also based on a Piagetian cognitive model. At the same time, the Nancy French approach also reflects the integration of Rorschach coding approaches of American and Canadian clinicians (Lerner, 1975, 1998; Schafer, 1954).

American Approaches

Unlike the European approaches, there is no contemporary holistic or integrated American system that governs how one would both administer and interpret the Rorschach and then link the findings to an underlying or overarching set of theoretical concepts that have special significance for understanding psychotic phenomena. The French and Swiss approaches can be thought of as holistic because they are not methodology-centered and do not focus narrowly on tests, but instead integrate tests, methods of administration, scoring, and interpretation into theoretically rich systems of personality structure and psychopathology.

From the 1930s through 1950s, Rorschach luminaries like Klopfer and Kelley (1942), Beck (1949), Hertz (1938), Piotrowski (1957), and Rapaport et al. (1968), mostly European immigrants themselves, developed separate systems of Rorschach administration and interpretation. These approaches existed in a parallel fashion, often vying for preeminence by criticizing the shortcomings of rival systems.

The Empirical Assessment of Psychotic Phenomena

Many approaches influenced by the Rapaport tradition focused more specifically on the Rorschach as a method for assessing psychotic phenomena. Although earlier American Rorschach contributors used the instrument to assess schizophrenia, one of Rapaport's major and enduring contributions to the Rorschach was his scores for deviant verbalizations (1968). Rapaport elevated the scores for deviant and disorganized language and illogical thinking to the level of a separate scoring dimension.

Two followers, Holt and Holzman, took Rapaport's scores for disordered thinking and developed empirically based scales for measuring deviant verbalization and illogical reasoning in Rorschach responses. Holt's PRIPRO (2009) is a comprehensive, yet time-consuming, instrument that has been used in countless studies since its inception (Holt, 1956). Holzman and colleagues developed the Thought Disorder Index (TDI; Holzman et al., 1986; Johnston & Holzman, 1979) as a tool for assessing forms of thought disorders. Although the TDI was initially also applied to verbalizations on the Wechlser Adult Intelligence Scale, it has been used primarily as a method for assessing disordered thinking on the Rorschach.

Comprehensive System and R-PAS
Between 1975 and 2010, except for small enclaves of clinicians who continued to use Klopfer or Rapaport, the Rorschach Comprehensive System (RCS) dominated the American Rorschach scene (Exner, 1974, 1986, 1993; Exner, Jr., 2003). Current American-based approaches, such as the RCS and the newer Rorschach Performance Assessment System (R-PAS; Meyer et al., 2011) have made substantial contributions to the development and survival of the Rorschach. Both are essentially atheoretical, single-instrument systems that are intended to focus only on a standardized and empirically supported method of Rorschach administration and interpretation. Just as the RCS was created from the most empirically robust bits and pieces of earlier American Rorschach systems, R-PAS was based only on those aspects of the RCS that have passed strict empirical muster (Mihura et al., 2013). Comparison of the systems has sparked a lively debate about the degree of overlap between the RCS and R-PAS (Mihura, 2019; Smith et al., 2018). Due largely to Mihura's meta-analytic studies (2013), R-PAS was used to score and interpret Peter's Rorschach.

Both the CS and R-PAS include individual scores and indices that pertain to dimensions relevant in the assessment of psychotic phenomena. Reality testing is largely assessed by the accuracy of form perception (Form Quality), and disturbances in thinking by a variety of scores and indices.

Inter-System Comparison of Peter's Rorschach

The idea of this collective paper emerged from a symposium on psychosis at the 2017 International Rorschach Congress in Paris. Clinicians representing three different Rorschach approaches analyzed Peter's Rorschach. Earlier, one of the members of the Nancy-French approach had administered the Rorschach to Peter at the end of a hospitalization. Peter had signed a written consent form agreeing to participate in a clinical case study. Each clinician on the panel had access to Peter's Rorschach, TAT, family background, and developmental history.

There were two reasons Peter was selected for this case study. First, the clinical team responsible for Peter's diagnosis and treatment disagreed about his diagnosis within the psychotic spectrum. Second, the complexity of the case suggested that a comparative analysis of the Rorschach test would be enlightening. Specifically, it was agreed that three separate Rorschach systems could help clarify whether Peter suffered from a paranoid psychosis (paranoia or delusional disorder) or paranoid schizophrenia.

For each studied dimension, we will analyze convergent and divergent points between our three approaches – see the tables and coding for each method in the Appendix.

Areas of Convergence

The three approaches reached similar interpretations on the following dimensions.

Nature of Conflict and Links to Reality

Each approach has used its own markers, codes, and scoring systems (different from one school to another) to point out Peter's severe reality impairment. For the Nancy approach, Rorschach indicators from the French coding system showed severe reality impairment, which was represented by the nature of the dominant conflicts between instincts and reality. According to the French approach (Chabert, 1983, 1987; de Tychey, 2012; Louët & Azoulay, 2016), in a psychotic mode, the conflict between instincts "*Ça*" (Id) and reality is represented by an increase in F% and a decrease in F+%. The French approach interprets elevated F% as a defensive attempt to cling to reality, as a way of screening out fantasies. At the same time, a decrease in F+% reflects the failure of this attempt among individuals within the psychotic spectrum. Peter clearly demonstrates these two signs with a very low F+% (11.8%) and a high F% (70%).

An additional score for the French approach is the Anxiety Indicator (IA%), which is the percentage of responses containing Hd+An+Sex+Bl. Peter's IA of 33% is considered highly pathological. This score signals a simultaneous burst of self-representation with a decompensation of the individual's psychotic personality organization. The two deteriorated popular responses (Pop) show the collapse of Peter's social adaptation.

There were similiarities in the conclusions of the Lausanne and R-PAS approaches. For the Lausanne approach, poor form responses have always been understood as a sign of poor reality testing. Peter starts his Rorschach with what Racamier (1980) has termed "hyperinterpretivity," in which the individual attributes inappropriate meaning to a response that is not grounded in the perceptual realities of the inkblot. For example, attributing qualities such as "wickedness" or referring to a "takeover" reflect hyperinterpretivity.

Speech coherence is another focus of concern for the Lausanne approach. Peter's speech was not always coherent and was occasionally difficult to understand. He also oscillated between affirmation and negation. This oscillation is viewed as a tolerance to contradiction, a phenomenon that is understood by Racamier as a sign of dissociation, where something and its opposite can simultaneously coexist in the self.

Two empirically robust R-PAS variables provide broad measures of psychopathology (Ego Impairment Index-3, EII-3, standard score = 143) and overall impairment in reality testing and thinking (Thought & Perception-Composite, TP-Comp, standard score = 142). As can be seen, Peter's standard scores on both measures reached the 99th percentile, indicating severity of psychopathology that most likely reached a psychotic level. More specific indices of reality testing demonstrated severe disturbance in Peter's abilities to separate his internal world from his perception of external stimuli. Minus Form Quality variables (FQ- and WD-%) were elevated beyond the 99th percentile, highlighting the severity of Peter's failure to form accurate impressions or critically evaluate the appropriateness of his perceptions. WD-% indicates that his reality testing is severely impaired even when he is responding to commonly perceived, easy-to-see location areas. His low scores tell us that he misses common cues that others often notice and he rarely forms accurate, conventional impressions. Collectively, these measures indicate that Peter's reality testing is severely compromised, making it unlikely that he can distinguish his thoughts and feelings from an objective appraisal of events and increasing the likelihood that he will form distorted impressions that do not comport with consensual reality.

Object Relations

In addition to identifying Rorschach indications of a symbiotic level of relatedness, the three approaches also noted features of Peter's paranoiac orientation. However, in their final diagnostic conclusions, each approach did not assign the same level of importance to these paranoiac features when they compared them with schizophrenic indicators.

The Nancy approach found indications of symbiosis in Peter's responses (e.g., note the theme of fusion in the first response to Card V). However, the authors identified persecution as the dominant form of Peter's object relations. Contrary to what can be observed in schizophrenia structures, where the object is merged with the subject, the objects depicted in Peter's responses are often distinct from the subject and characterized by a persecutory paranoid mode. This same persecutory quality was also reflected in Peter's interactions with the examiner. The examiner's questions appeared to systematically trigger the projection of mistrust and malevolent intentionality typical of paranoiacs. For example, Peter's first comment on Card I was, "What's the point of all these tests I'm taking? To trap me?" Similarly, on Card VI, Peter revealed his persecutory mindset with his comment,"You see people laughing, I feel like they are making fun of me." The Nancy approach noted the same potential fantasized interactions in his response R1, "wickedness, the severe eyes"; R2, "Wickedness, really, perceptible evil, and a smile like that, not vicious, a mean smile"; and R21, "It looks like a human stare or a tiger who is watching you and who's sulking." This suggests that Peter was poised to perceive the environment as an external threat from the first (cf. R1) to the last card (cf. R24). The analysis of intrapsychic functioning in terms of representations of object relations thus makes it possible to understand the permanence of Peter's paranoid symptomatology in terms of his clinical behavior.

Another indicator of Peter's dominant paranoiac orientation for the Nancy approach was the frequency of responses reflecting an "Anal Perspective." We used Schafer's (1954) qualitative criteria for the definition of Anal Perspective. For example, the projection of the fantasy of anal penetration (see Card 2 R5: "And there, it looks like a penis which is going to penetrate a man"), emphasizes the importance of a homosexual, anal preoccupation specific to paranoiac functioning, a finding consistent with this theoretical model.

For the Lausanne approach, symbiosis is anxiety provoking, as it presents a risk of engulfment into the other and, as such, rapprochement often generates feelings of persecution. For Peter, the examiner clearly exists. There are many occasions on which he calls upon the examiner ("you know"). These formulations can represent attempts to establish a symbiosis of thought, that is, to make sure that the examiner thinks the same as the speaker. Symbiosis is also manifest in the belief that both parties share the same experience. For example, on Card III, Peter said, "It feels like *we* can't escape from an enclosed space." The "we" in his comment includes the examiner in an anxiety-provoking situation, laden with persecution emanating from some obscure source or unknown force. The threat is, at times, explicitly verbalized, as when Peter asked suspiciously on Card I, "What's the point of all these tests I'm taking? To trap me?" This clearly illustrates how the relationship with object (here, the examiner) is of a persecutory nature. The fantasy of being trapped is central to personalities with traits of paranoia.

The R-PAS variable NPH/SumH (Non-Pure H Proportion) was clinically significant (standard score 122). This ratio compares the number of human details, or Hd, and fantasized human, (H) and (Hd), to the number of pure human contents, H. Peter's significant NPH/SumH showed a preponderance of human details or fantasized human responses, reflecting a more primitive part-object orientation. From this vantage point, Peter does not perceive others as whole, integrated figures, but as fragmented parts and functions lacking in breadth and depth. Peter only gave one full human response on Card V. Although the form quality was ordinary, the response itself, "a man who moves his wings," was illogical.

His other Rorschach scores pertaining to object representations include Human Movement Form Quality minus (M-, Standard Score 123), Mutuality of Autonomy–Pathology/Mutuality of Autonomy–Health (MAP/MAH, Standard Score 123), Poor Human Representation/Good + Poor Human Representation (PHR/GPHR, standard score 133), Space Reversal (SR, standard score 122), Uncommon Detail (Dd%, standard score 118), and Vigilance Composite (V-Comp, standard score 118). Collectively, these scores capture Peter's (1) misunderstanding of others' thoughts and intentions (elevated number of Human Movement, poor form quality, or M-, responses), (2) attribution of malevolent and threatening intent and relating to others in maladaptive ways (clinically significant MAP/MAH, PHR/GPHR), (3) resistance to control, and (4) tendency to focus on small and idiosyncratic details with an effortful, guarded, and suspicious cognitive style (SR, Dd%, V-Comp). Together, these variables define distinct structural characteristics of a paranoid style.

Self-Representation and Anxiety

The three approaches interpreted many variables pertaining to self-representation and anxiety similarly. For example, the Nancy approach noted the limited number of whole, accurately perceived human and animal responses and the low ratio of whole to partial human and animal responses, which might suggest a schizophrenic fragmentation of self-representation. Although fragmented contents were present (see very pathological IA% of 33%), the Nancy clinicians did not view this as schizophrenic fragmentation anxiety, because Peter's dominant anxiety appeared more related to fragmentation precipitated by a fear of anal penetration. For example, his responses on Card II were seen as graphic depictions of anal penetration anxiety. Peter's undisguised preoccupation with anal penetration was followed abruptly by a defensive reference to putting on a hat. Not only was his reference to "putting on a hat" loose and obscure, but it also did not fend off the emotional charge from his previous anal content, which re-emerged at the end of his response. The Nancy approach also noted how Peter grimaced as he ended his responses to Card II and added, "That male organ, yuck." His Response 12 on Card V reflects this same degree of anguish, although in a slightly less symbolic way.

The Lausanne approach found various examples of vague and ill-defined identity or sense of self, such as "a *sort* of face" (Card II); "*someone* who imposes himself" (Card IV); and "a *human being*" (Card IX). Other responses reflected partial or fragmented representations of the disembodied body parts, such as "severe eyes" (Card I); "a smile" (Card I); "no eyes, no mouth, no nose... an expression" (Card II); and "a penis which is going to penetrate a man" (Card II). A number of these body parts carry intentions of their own, as if they were the whole person.

Regarding drives, Peter's responses contained ample sexual contents and scenarios. The Lausanne approach noted how his sexual responses reflected crude and uncensored fantasies. They also saw the significance of the theme of anality, which was clearly present in several responses, including the image of "a penis which is going to penetrate a man" at Card II. Other responses reflected percepts seen from behind. For example, Peter saw Card IV as "a rooster with a very red neck... (Inquiry) it also looks like we are seeing it from behind," and Card V as "an animal *taken* from behind." Preoccupation with objects seen from behind is consistent with persecutory anxieties about what might be happening behind one's back.

Peter's protocol contains different levels of anxiety. Some contents reflect an interest in occult forces, such as "wickedness" seen in Card I or the "demons" in Card X, which were not associated with specific objects. The "severe eyes" that he saw on Card I were fragmented body parts, which supported the idea of fragmentation anxiety. At times, Peter focused his anxiety on a defined persecutor such as the examiner. As noted earlier, his anxiety regarding anal penetration was clearly evident in the graphic response on Card II of "a penis which is going to penetrate a man." The anxiety of anal penetration is obvious but the fragmentation is also apparent in that he refers to a penis, that is, a body part in action. Peter was also preoccupied with the eyes, and the acts of looking and staring. The Lausanne approach viewed these references as signs of paranoid anxiety, a form of persecution that is more archaic than the one encountered in paranoiacs who succeed in crystallizing their anxiety onto defined people.

R-PAS variables pertaining to Self and Other Representations highlight his experience of threat and vulnerability. Elevated MAP/MAHP and anatomy content (An) capture his threatened and vulnerable sense of self. His Card VIII response of an "opened human body" vividly reflects this vulnerability and exposure. A significant Vigilance Composite (V-Comp) represents a guarded, self-protective stance, as the content of his responses reveal heightened perceptions of penetration, dominance, and external control. Yet, despite his vigilance and vulnerability to attack, Peter does not appear to experience the affective upheaval that his sense of external threat would lead us to expect. None of the R-PAS Stress and Distress variables are clinically significant, suggesting an absence of anguish and turmoil. Thus, his vigilance against external threats and malevolence seems to have a self-protective function and to have lowered his level of palpable anguish.

Defense Mechanisms

Clinicians' interpretations converged in their analysis of Peter's dominant defense mechanisms. Beginning with the Nancy approach, clinicians followed Lerner's suggestion (1975, 1998) to code the most frequently used defense mechanisms. To code all primitive defense mechanisms, we used French qualitative definition criteria elaborated by Chabert (1983, 1987), and completed by Louët and Azoulay (2016), and Anglo-Saxon qualitative definition criteria suggested by Schafer (1954) and Lerner (1975, 1998; see Appendix). Peter's primitive defenses indicate a psychotic level of functioning. More specifically, his reponses suggest splitting, projection and projective identification, denial of reality, and duplication of the ego. For example, splitting may be represented by the deteriorated and confabulated verbalization of R6 ("There, it looks like a skull with glasses, right there") and associated with the projection in his R2 response ("Wickedness, really, perceptible evil, and a smile like that, not vicious, a mean smile"). The denial of reality is already inferable from the global collapse of any sense of reality (cf. F+%, 11.8%). This denial takes on near delusional proportions when compared with the symbolism of the phallic power of Card 4, where Peter sees the color red in an entirely black card (cf. R10: "An animal ... A rooster with a very red neck"). The dissociation of the ego may be reflected in Peter's Card VII R17 response, "Ah, there are two small persons, a baby with a tail," which depicts a condensation of human and animal features.

The projection suggested by several of Peter's fragmented responses of partial human and degraded animal responses (e.g., R14, R15, R18) has a distinct persecutory quality. The paranoiac dimension present in many responses is characteristic of a paranoid psychotic structure. This structure represents a central component in the dynamics of Peter's intrapsychic functioning and is apparent throughout his responses (e.g., R1, R2, R3, R4, R7, R13, R21, R22, R24). The defense of projective identification, suggested by Peter's tendency to expel and attribute internalized negativity to external objects, infiltrates many of his responses (cf. R1, R2, R3, and other small kinesthesic with aggressive valence). Finally, his frequent reference to the eyes (four times in the protocol) reflects, according to Schafer (1954), the hypervigilance of the paranoiac with respect to the outside world.

For the Lausanne approach, projection of evil or malevolent intent was reflected in responses such as, a "mean smile," "absolute evil," or reference to how the test was "to trap me." Denial of reality takes the form of color projection in Peter's response on Card IV of "a rooster with a very red neck" and on Card III "a skull with glasses". The group adhered to Pasche's (1982) definition of projective identification whereby the bad object is projected onto an external source and then comes back to the subject like a boomerang. This process is reflected in the verbalization, "It looks like a human stare or a tiger who is watching you."

Finally, the R-PAS notes how Peter maintains a vigilant and protective stance against external threats. Significant elevations on M-, Dd, and V-Comp reflect a dominant use of projective mechanisms to reduce his anxiety. He surveys small idiosyncratic details and forms inaccurate impressions of others and their actions and motivations. Unfortunately, his reduction in anxiety and anguish comes at a high cost – a highly distorted picture of others.

Disordered Thinking

This last dimension does not have the same relevance in specifying personality organization for the three approaches, although they all recognized the severity of Peter's disordered thought processes in his Rorschach protocol.

The Nancy approach identified a severe level of thought disorder in Peter's protocol (coded in the Parisian approach by confabulations and contaminations). Such a degree of severity in thought organization might suggest a structure within the schizophrenic spectrum. However, the Nancy clinicians did not come to this conclusion, because Bergeret did not view markers of cognitive functioning as constants in differential diagnostic decision-making. It should also be noted that, in Bergeret's theoretical model (1974, 1986), it is the primitivity of defense mechanisms that are responsible for both delusions, verbalized in the interviews (see anamnesis), and disordered thinking (represented by confabulations, contaminations) projected in the representation of reality through the Rorschach test.

The Lausanne approach uses Racamier's concept of *hyperinterpretivity* where, basically, the individual puts too much meaning into the blot: "wickedness," a "takeover" (1966). Peter's speech is often confused and incoherent. His tolerance to contradiction can be understood as a sign of dissociation, since something and its opposite can coexist in the self simultaneously. Dissociation in Bergeret's model is a sign of a splitting of the self (*dédoublement du Moi*) and fits with the scission described by Bleuler (1911/1993) in schizophrenia. A number of confabulations are to be underlined: "a skull with glasses," "an animal, a man who opens his wings," "a baby with a tail."

Disordered thinking is an important focus in American Rorschach traditions. The R-PAS variable WSumCog (Weighted Sum of Six Cognitive Codes) focuses more narrowly on pervasiveness of disturbed thinking, while SevCog (Severe Cognitive Codes) addresses the severity of the disturbance. All of Peter's scores are clinically significant and reflect severe impairment in the qualities of his thinking. Regarding the concept of disturbed thinking, or thought disorder, it is useful to distinguish between disorganized and illogical thought processes

(Kleiger, 2017). Disorganization is characterized by disruptions in communication. The speaker has difficulties focusing, filtering, ordering, and sequencing thought as expressed through speech. As a result, the listener is often confused about what the speaker is trying to convey. Rorschach scores reflecting disorganization include Deviant Verbalizations (DV) and associative-Deviant Responses (DR). In DVs and DRs, communication is disrupted at the level of individual words and expressions. The speaker uses language that departs from conventional usage, leaving the listener at a loss to fully comprehend the speaker's intended meaning.

Whereas *disorganization* pertains to how something is said, *illogicality* has to do with the quality of the person's reasoning about what it is they say. Typically, illogical Rorschach responses are classified as (1) combinatory (FABs or fabulized combinations and INCs or incongruous combinations), (2) confabulatory (interpretative-DRs, in which the speaker embellishes the response with inappropriate detail, attributions, or specificity), and (3) autistic or peculiar logic (ALOG in CS and PEC in R-PAS, where the speaker explicitly bases his/her conclusions on a peripheral detail). Illogical responses (INC, FAB, and DR) can also be designated as either Level 1 or Level 2 severity, depending upon the degree of logical departure and bizarreness.

Peter demonstrated both qualities of disturbance in his Rorschach responses. First with the Rorschach, he had three Level-2 DRs (DR2, standard score 142) on Cards III, V, and VI and a Level-2 FAB (standard score 127) on Card III. Peter first saw Card III as a "skull with glasses," which reflects a milder form of illogicality. Skulls with glasses are not impossible, but they are quite improbable. However, his second response involved a more bizarre and patently illogical combination of images. It also concluded with a cryptic comment that made little sense.

It looks like women's underwear...and there, it seems, a taking of control with respect to the skull [FAB2]...Like absolute evil with (shows the takeover with his hands). It feels like we can't escape from an enclosed space [DR2]... I don't see how any of this is useful for you...

Concluding Remarks

It is interesting to note that, although the three approaches agreed regarding the numerous signs of psychotic functioning, they differed in their interpretation of these signs. The key difference was in terms of whether Peter's personality structure was best understood as paranoiac or schizophrenic in nature. The Nancy approach interpretation viewed Peter's underlying personality structure as paranoiac. Like the Lausanne approach, the R-PAS approach interpretation agreed that Peter's impairment was more characteristic of a predominantly schizophrenic (paranoid schizophrenia) than a paranoid disturbance or structure.

Despite agreeing that Peter's psychological functioning was organized at a psychotic level, the Nancy approach interpretation does not view the primary diagnosis as schizophrenia. Their conclusions were centered solely on Bergeret's theoretical model, in which interpretation is based on the frequency of intrapsychic constants specific to each type of psychopathology. Contrary to the Lausanne and American approaches, little attention is given to disorders of thinking. As noted earlier, even though there were several examples of disordered thinking in Peter's protocol, Bergeret believed that cognitive functioning is altered in all modes of psychotic organization. The nature and number of thought disorders depend in part on the degree of decompensation of the individual's structural organization, on the defensive mechanisms that they will use at the time of their decompensation, and on the influence of the neuroleptic medication administered, which is not without consequences on the functioning of the person's thought process and the type of disorders that he or she will or will not continue to display.

When two or more different signs belonging to different intrapsychic organizations are present (as is the case here), Bergeret recommended scoring the most frequent of them because they identify the structure of intrapsychic functionning. Thus, according to this model, Nancy clinicians felt that it was reasonable to conclude that the dominant feature of Peter's intrapsychic functioning was paranoiac in nature.

Despite his severely disordered thinking and delusional core, it is important to note that Peter now lives outside of the hospital setting and had maintained a relatively adequate external adaptation. The latter feature has rendered the creation of a therapeutic alliance difficult, although not impossible, due to the constant projection of mistrust and malicious intentionality that saturate most of his relationships.

Contrary to the conclusions of the Nancy group, both the Lausanne and American approaches viewed Peter's underlying disturbance to be of a paranoid schizophrenic nature. For the Lausanne approach, this was apparent in his fragmented self, overwhelming paranoid anxiety, poor reality testing, and clear presence of disordered thinking and perplexity. Peter appeared to lose distance when responding to the cards and to embue the contents of his responses as animated and threatening. At times Peter circumscribed his anxiety and projected it onto a defined persecutor, such as the examiner and the people in the next room. His preoccupation with anal penetration is distinct and different from the usual fantasies of oral aggressivity often present in paranoid schizophrenics.

The Lausanne approach has a more integrative approach: It relies on Bergeret's model but it is also influenced by other psychoanalytic and cognitive models and gives more attention to cognitive markers to make a distinction between paranoid psychosis (paranoia) and paranoid schizophrenic psychosis. Here the clinician (as does the American clinician) chooses to prioritize cognitive markers to differentiate the two organizations. The Lausanne approach viewed Peter's paranoiac defenses as protective in nature, helping him avoid a more florid schizophrenic presentation. Racamier (1966) proposed the concept of *schizoparanoia* for individuals who are fundamentally schizophrenic but who construct such paranoiac defenses. By contrast, paranoiacs tend not to hear voices and their delusions sound more plausible and convincing, whereas Peter's delusions are improbable with no clearly defined persecutor. As a result, the Lausanne clinician concluded that Peter suffered from schizophrenia. Had he been a true paranoiac, he would have been less treatable because of an even heightened suspicion.

From a contemporary American perspective, Peter's testing is consistent with disturbances in thinking and reality testing, which are likely to have reached a psychotic level of severity. Concluding that Peter was actively psychotic at the time of his evaluation would be strongly supported by the testing evidence. There is also a convergence of indicators of paranoid dynamics, supported by formal features of the testing and ample themes of threat, mistrust, sadomasochism, vulnerability, and penetration.

There is ample evidence in Peter's testing of fixed paranoid themes and formal scores characteristic of paranoid dynamics. However, the extent of conceptual disorganization was unmistakable. He not only suffered from severe paranoia, but Peter's thinking could also become loose and disorganized. Diagnostically, this shifts our understanding to the realm of schizophrenia and would lead us to conclude that he was suffering from paranoid schizophrenia, as opposed to a more circumscribed paranoid or delusional disorder.

It is clear that the relative significance of theoretical versus empirical factors differed in each of the schools or traditions. The conclusions of the Nancy French approach are based on a single theoretical model. By contrast, the Lausanne and American approaches use several models and empirical data to enable clinicians to integrate theoretical and/or empirical markers to advance diagnostic conclusions. Compared to the other two approaches, the American approach is conceptually leaner and more economical in terms of reliance on underlying theoretical models to support diagnostic inferences. In analyzing Peter's Rorschach, the American approach would focus more narrowly on ego functioning, specifically the nature of reality testing and disturbances in thinking, as opposed to dominant anxiety, defenses, object relations, boundaries, and libidinal issues. Here, the focus is on the nature of the disturbance in thinking, which may involve disorganization of thought processes and speech, on the one hand, and a breakdown in logic, on the other.

Limitations of the Case Study Method

There are numerous limitations in our presentation of different approaches to interpreting Peter's testing data. First, for practical reasons having to do with manuscript length, we have only presented Peter's Rorschach data. The Nancy approach integrates scores from the Rorschach and the MMPI-2-RF for clinical diagnosis, and the Lausanne approach always relies on material both from the Rorschach and TAT. American approaches advocate multimethod assessment that includes performance-based methods along with self-report inventories.

Additionally, we lack longitudinal testing data that would have helped determine Peter's functioning over time. Re-testing him at a latter point might have revealed which components of his intrapsychic world were more entrenched and which might have responded to treatment.

References

American Psychiatric Association (2013). *Diagnostic and statistical manual of mental disorders* (5th ed.).

Barthes, R. (1980). *La chambre claire* [The clear room]. Gallimard.

Beck, S. (1949). *Rorschach's test, Vol. 1: Basic processes* (2nd ed). Grune & Stratton.

Bergeret, J. (1974). *La personnalité normale et pathologique* [Normal and pathological personality]. Dunod.

Bergeret, J. (1986). *Abrégés de Psychopathologie* [Abstract of psychopathology]. Masson. (Original work published 1911)

Bleuler, E. (1993). *Dementia praecox ou groupe des schizophrénies* [Dementia praecox or schizophrenia group]. Éditions E.P.E.L (Original work published 1955).

Bohm, E. (1985). *Traité du psychodiagnostic de Rorschach* [Rorschach Psychodiagnostic Manual]. Masson.

Chabert, C. (1983). *Le Rorschach en clinique adulte: Interpretation psychanalytique* [The Rorschach in adult clinical settings: Psychoanalytic interpretation]. Dunod.

Chabert, C. (1987). *La Psychopathologie à travers le Rorschach* [Psychopathology throughout the Rorschach]. Dunod.

De Tychey, C. (2012). *Le Rorschach en clinique de la dépression adulte* [Rorschach test in adult clinical depression field]. Dunod.

Exner, J. E. (1974). *The Rorschach: A comprehensive system* (Vol. 1). Wiley.

Exner, J. E. (1986). *The Rorschach: A comprehensive system* (2nd ed., Vol. 1). Wiley.

Exner, J. E. (1993). *The Rorschach: A comprehensive system* (3rd ed., Vol. 1). Wiley.

Exner, J. E. Jr. (2003). *The Rorschach: A comprehensive system* (4th ed.). Wiley.

Rorschachiana (2022), 43(1), 42–69

Hertz, M. R. (1938). Scoring the Rorschach ink-blot test. *Journal of Genetic Psychology, 52,* 15–64.

Holt, R. (2009). *Primary process thinking: Theory, measurement, and research* (Vols. 1 & 2). Aronson.

Holt, R. R. (1956). Gauging primary and secondary process in Rorschach responses. *Journal of Projective Techniques,* 20, 14–25..

Holzman, P. E., Shenton, M. E., & Solovay, M. R. (1986). Quality of thought disorder in differential diagnosis. *Schizophrenia Bulletin, 12,* 360–371.

Johnston, M. H., & Holzman, P. S. (1979). *Assessing schizophrenic thinking.* Jossey-Bass.

Kleiger, J. H. (2017). *Rorschach assessment of psychotic phenomena: Clinical, conceptual, and empirical developments.* Taylor & Francis.

Klopfer, B., & Kelley, D. M. (1942). *The Rorschach technique: A manual for a projective method of personality diagnosis.* World Book Company.

Lerner, P. M. (1975). *Handbook of Rorschach scales.* International Universities Press.

Lerner, P. M. (1998). *Psychoanalytic perspectives on the Rorschach.* The Analytic Press.

Louët, E., & Azoulay, C. (2016). *Schizophrénie et paranoïa: Étude psychanalytique en clinique projective* [Schizophrenia and paranoia: A psychoanalytic clinical and projective study]. Dunod.

Meyer, G. J., Viglione, D. J., Mihura, J. L., Erard, R. E., & Erdberg, P. (2011). *Rorschach Performance Assessment System: Administration, coding, interpretation, and technical manual.* Rorschach Performance Assessment System.

Mihura, J. L. (2019). Correcting Smith et al.'s (2018) criticisms of all Rorschach studies in Mihura, Meyer, Dumitrascu, and Bombel's (2013) meta-analyses. *Rorschachiana, 40*(2), 169–186. https://doi.org/10.1027/1192-5604/a000118

Mihura, J. L., Meyer, G. J., Dumitrascu, N., & Bombel, G. (2013). The validity of individual Rorschach variables: Systematic reviews and meta-analyses of the comprehensive system. *Psychological Bulletin, 139*(3), 548–605.

Pasche, F. (1982). À propos de l'identification projective [About projective identification]. *Revue française de psychanalyse, 46*(2), 408–411.

Piaget, J., & Inhelder, B. (1966). *La psychologie de l'enfant* [Child psychology]. PUF.

Piotrowski, Z. A. (1957). *Perceptanalysis.* Macmillan.

Racamier, P. C. (1966). Esquisse d'une clinique psychanalytique de la paranoïa [Sketch of a psychoanalytic clinic of paranoïa]. *Revue française de psychanalyse, 30*(1), 145–172.

Racamier, P. C. (1980). *Les schizophrènes* [Schizophrenic patients]. Payot.

Rapaport, D., Gill, M., & Schafer, R. (1968). *Diagnostic psychological testing* (revised ed.). International Universities Press.

Schafer, R. (1954). *Psychoanalytic interpretation in Rorschach testing.* Grune & Stratton.

Smith, J. M., Gacono, C. B., Fontan, P., Taylor, E. E., Cunliffe, T. B., & Andronikof, A. (2018). A scientific critique of Rorschach research: Revisiting Exner's Issues and Methods in Rorschach Research (1995). *Rorschachiana, 39*(2), 180–203. https://doi.org/10.1027/1192-5604/a000102

History
Received March 5, 2019
Revision received June 21, 2021
Accepted July 13, 2021
Published online April 28, 2022

Publication Ethics

The name of the patient has been anonymized. The authors have written consent from the patient agreeing to participate in a clinical case study.

Cécile Prudent
Private Practice
31 Avenue Colgate
13009 Marseille
France
cecile.prudent@gmail.com

Summary

This article emerged from a symposium that focused on psychosis at the last International Rorschach Congress held in Paris in 2017. The authors are doctoral-level clinicians representing three different Rorschach approaches or systems. The author independently coded and analyzed the Rorschach data of a patient called "Peter," in a triple-blind procedure. One clinician used the Rorschach Performance Assessment System (R-PAS), developed by American psychologists. Another followed the Lausanne Rorschach approach and the others represented the Nancy subgroup of Parisian systems. Each clinician author was given the same background information related to the patient's clinical anamnesis. Peter had been selected because his clinical hospital, in charge of making a diagnosis and providing treatment, had disagreed about where to place him diagnostically on the psychotic spectrum. For example, some felt the diagnosis should be paranoid psychosis, while others thought that either a delusional disorder or paranoid schizophrenia were more accurate diagnoses of Peter's psychotic-level disorder.

The authors first present the background of their three approaches from varying theoretical and clinical points of view. The Rorschach coding and interpretation are based on French psychoanalytical, American R-PAS, and Canadian Lausanne conceptualizations. The diagnostic conclusions of the Nancy French group are based primarily on Bergeret's single theoretical model completed with American (Schafer) and Canadian (Lerner) psychoanalytical coding propositions. By contrast, the Lausanne group has a more integrative approach, which includes Bergeret's model, but it is also influenced by other psychoanalytical, cognitive (e.g., Piaget), and linguistic (e.g., Barthes) models, as well. The American approach focuses primarily on the empirically based Rorschach Performance Assessment System (R-PAS), with particular emphasis on disturbances in thinking and perception associated with psychotic-level disorders.

Comparative analyses show many convergent points between clinicians based on five dimensions (nature of conflicts and links to reality, object relations, self-representation and anguish, defensive dominant mechanisms, and thought disorders). However, the diagnostic conclusions are slightly different (paranoid psychosis for Nancy, schizo-paranoia for Lausanne, and paranoid schizophrenia based primarily on R-PAS). The main explanation for their differences is related to the fact the Nancy French group's diagnostic conclusions are centered on Bergeret's single structural model. Inside this model, interpretation is based on occurrence of intrapsychic constants specific to each psychopathology. In contrast to the American and Lausanne approaches, the Nancy group devotes less attention to disorders of thinking. Instead, the Nancy integrative approach focuses more on the cognitive markers to make the distinction between paranoid psychosis and paranoid schizophrenic psychosis.

Résumé

Cet article a émergé d'un symposium sur les psychoses lors du dernier congrès international du Rorschach. Le Rorschach fut analysé séparément, en triple aveugle, par chaque membre de trois écoles (deux cliniciens du groupe de Nancy appartenant à l'Ecole de Paris, un clinicien américain et un du Groupe de Lausanne).

La même information reliée au cas clinique (Peter 37 ans) a été donnée à chacun. Le patient a été sélectionné parce que l'équipe hospitalière responsable du diagnostic et du traitement était en désaccord sur le diagnostic dans le spectre psychotique (psychose paranoïde [paranoïa ou trouble délirant] ou schizophrénie paranoïde?).

Les auteurs présentent d'abord les caractéristiques différentes des trois groupes sur le plan de leurs modèles théorico-cliniques de référence. Le Groupe de Nancy est monocentré sur la théorie psychanalytique structurale de Bergeret. La codification et l'interprétation des données Rorschach dans une perspective psychanalytique s'appuie à la fois sur les apports de l'Ecole de Paris et les conceptualisations psychanalytiques anglo-saxonnes américaines (Schafer) et canadiennes (Lerner). Le Groupe de Lausanne a une perspective intégrative sur le plan théorique avec des références plurielles sur le plan psychanalytique (Bergeret, Racamier) associées à des références cognitives piagétiennes et linguistiques (Barthes). Les écoles américaines actuelles avec le R-PAS ont accordé plus d'attention au soubassement empirique des variables Rorschach et ont fondé leur sélection et interprétation des variables Rorschach sur des résultats de recherche davantage centrés sur le niveau cognitif des troubles de la pensée.

Les données analysées ont mis en évidence les points de convergence entre les trois groupes pour attester du fonctionnement psychotique de Peter sur 5 dimensions importantes pour le diagnostic: la nature des conflits et les liens à la réalité, les relations d'objet, la représentation de soi et l'angoisse, les mécanismes de défense dominants et les troubles de la pensée. Mais le cadre de référence théorico-clinique différent de chaque groupe conduit à une interprétation diagnostique légèrement différente : l'approche Américaine et de Lausanne concluent à un diagnostic de sujet schizoparanoïde ou de schizoparanoïa et le Groupe de Nancy à un diagnostic de psychose paranoïaque. La raison principale de ces divergences est liée au fait que les deux premiers groupes, dans leur hiérarchie des facteurs diagnostiques, privilégient les facteurs cognitifs liés aux troubles de la pensée alors que le groupe nancéen, à partir du modèle de Bergeret, privilégie les constantes structurales du fonctionnement intrapsychique, sans donner aux troubles cognitifs la même importance.

Resumen

Este articulo emergió de un simposio sobre psicosis durante el ultimo congreso International del Rorschach en Paris. El protocolo de Rorschach fuera analizó separadamente por tres especialistas (dos psicólogos clínicos del grupo de Nancy que pertenecen a la escuela de Paris, un estado americano y otro de la escuela suiza de Lausanne).

La misma información conectado al caso clínico (Peter 37 años), se le dio a cada uno. El paciente fuera seleccionado porque el equipo del hospital responsable del diagnostico y del tratamiento era ene desacuerdo en este por d'entro del espectro psicótico (paranoide psicosis o esquizofrenia paranoide).

Autores presentan primero las diferentes características de los tres grupos sobre el plan theorico-clínico de referencia. El grupo de Nancy esta centrado sobre la teoría psicoanalítica estructuralista de Jean Bergeret. La codificación y la interpretación de los datos Rorschach en esta perspectiva se confía a la vez sobre la contribuciones de la escuela de Paris y sobre la conceptualización de

Schafer (Estado-americano) y de Lerner (Canadian). La escuela de Lausanne tiene una perspectiva integrativa con referencias plurales en el plano psicoanalítico (Bergeret, Racamier) asociadas a referencias cognitiva de Piaget. La escuela americana actual with Comprehensive Sysytem and R-Pas han concedido mas importancia al sótano empírico de las variables Rorschach y fundado su selección y interpretación desee sobre los resultados de las investigaciones más centradas sobre el nivel cognitiva de las alteraciones del pensamiento.

Los datos analizados ponen en evidencia el punto de convergencia entre los tres grupos para atestar del modo de funcionamiento psicótico de Peter en sus 5 dimensiones importantes por el diagnostico: la natura del conflicto y los enlaces a la realidad, el tipo de relacionamiento del objeto, la autorrepresentación y el nivel de la angustia, los mecanismos de defensas y las alteraciones del pensamiento. Pero el cuadro de referencia teórica es diferente por cada escuela con diagnósticos diferentes de psicosis. La razón principal de este diferencias tiene a la jerarquización de los factores diagnosticas. Los dos primeras grupos privilegian factores sobre las alteraciones de los pensamientos cuando el grupo de Nancy prefiere privilegiar las constantes estructuralistas de la operación intrapsíquica.

要約

この論文は、2017年に開催された国際ロールシャッハ及び投映法学会のパリ大会にて、精神病に焦点を当てたシンポジウムから生まれたものである。筆者は、"ピーター"と呼ばれる患者のロールシャッハデータを、三重盲検法で独自にコードし分析した。一人の臨床家は、アメリカの心理学者によって開発されたR-PASを使用し、もう一人は、ローザンヌ・ロールシャッハ法を用い、他の一人はパリ法ナンシーサブグループを代表するシステムを使用した。それぞれの臨床家には、患者の既往歴に関する背景情報が伝えられた。今回ピーターが選ばれたのは、彼を診断し治療をしていた病院で、彼を精神病スペクトラムのどこに位置づけるかについて、意見が分かれたからである。例えば、妄想性精神病を診断すべきだと考える人もいれば、妄想性障害または妄想型統合失調症のどちらかがピーターを診断する上でより正確であると考える人もいた。

筆者らはまず、理論的・臨床的観点の異なる3つのアプローチの背景を提示する。ロールシャッハのコーディングと解釈は、フランスの精神分析的理論、アメリカのR-PAS、カナダのローザンヌの概念に基づいている。ナンシー・フランチグループの診断結果は、主にアメリカ（Schafer）とカナダ（Lerner）の精神分析的コーディングからなるベルジェットの単一の理論モデルに基づいている。これに対し、ローザンヌグループは、ベルジェットのモデルを含みながらも、他の精神分析的なモデルや認知モデル（ピアジェなど）、言語モデル（バルトなど）にも影響を受けている。アメリカのアプローチは、主に経験則に基づいたR-PASに焦点をあて、特に精神病レベルの障害における思考と知覚の障害に重きを置いている。

比較分析では、5つの側面（葛藤の本質と現実との関連、対象との関係、自己表象と苦悩、防衛的支配メカニズム、思考障害）に基づいて、臨床家の間で多くの収束点が示されている。しかし、診断上の結論は若干異なっている（ナンシーは妄想性障害、ローザンヌは統合失調-パラノイア、R-PASは妄想型統合失調症）。その主な理由は、ナンシー・フレンチグループが診断をする際にベルジェットの単一構造モデルに重きを置いていることに関連している。このモデルでは、それぞれの精神病理学に特異的な精神内部の発生に基づいて解釈がなされる。アメリカやローザンヌのアプローチとは対照的に、ナンシーグループは思考の障害にあまり注意を払わない。その代わり、ナンシー統合アプローチでは、妄想性障害と妄想型統合失調症を区別するために、認知マーカーにより重点を置いている。

Appendix A

Peter's Background History (Anamnesis)

The clinical case chosen for this study is a 37-year-old man whom we call "Peter." The Nancy School clinicians selected Peter for this case study because they had consulted with his medical team and felt that his symptoms raised diagnostic issues about whether paranoiac personality disorders should be included in the psychotic spectrum.

Diagnosed with paranoid schizophrenia at the end of his adolescence, Peter lives with a tyrannical voice that prevents him from leading a very ordered life. Peter's diet, for instance, is governed by this voice. To appease his suffering, he undergoes regular antipsychotic treatments (one tablet in the morning and one in the afternoon).

Raised in a family of lawyers, Peter is the oldest of three children. The two other brothers are married. Peter graduated from the university and worked in marketing but is now on long-term sick leave. Peter lives a relatively structured life. He wakes up early and goes to bed late. Every day, he walks for 1 hr. His relationship with his parents, with whom he has always lived, is generally harmonious; however, he fears criticism from his father, who has not always been kind to him or his brothers. His father was absent during their childhood, and Peter remembers feeling frightened when he heard his father's footsteps on the stairs of the family house. By contrast, he describes his mother as a much easier parent.

Peter demonstrated a degree of insight when he commented, "It did me good to return to X [a psychiatric hospital]. It was paradise. I walked in the parking lot, and I saw a person, and I said to myself, 'That is God'." Despite his apparent awareness of his illness and need for treatment, his persistent auditory hallucinations still prevent him from speaking about certain things. For example, he is convinced that there is a conspiracy against him, and, if he speaks about it, his voices will turn on him.

At first, it was difficult to establish a bond with Peter because of his paranoia, but he soon learned to trust us (i.e., one of the authors of this article who was also Peter's therapist) and appreciated our sessions together. We had to contain him psychically and not be intrusive because he felt threatened and feared that his voices will reproach him or make him pay for his denunciations. Although at the end of our interviews he confided a lot, he seemed to appease his voices by stating: "I did not reveal anything; no one can accuse me."

It is extremely difficult to place Peter in relation to traditional psychiatric and psychoanalytical diagnostic systems. In the DSM-5, Peter received a diagnosis of delusional disorder (297.1; ICD-10, F22). We could not make the diagnosis of paranoid personality disorder (301.0; ICD-10, F60.0; American Psychiatric

Association, 2013, p. 764, in the French translation, 2015) because that diagnosis appears in psychotic disorders (entry DSM-5) and in schizophrenia (entry DSM-IV-R) and is excluded by Criterion B (American Psychiatric Association, 2013, p. 764).

The favorite card: This one is ugly, no? This one here is pretty (10) because there's lots of colors.
The card least liked: 9
The card that most resembles you: Um, none
The card that most resembles your father: Oh no, let's not talk about my father
The card that most resembles your mother: 10

Structural Summary
R = 24; Total Time = 1900"; T/R= 190"; TL mean = 24,5"
1 WS; 1 DW; 6 W-; SumG% = 32; G+% = 0
Sum D% = 56%; Sum Dd% = 12%; Sum S% = 8,33%
Succession = 3 : (P2, P7, P8) : incoherent TA: G-D- *dbl-Dd*
F%[1]= 15 F- et 2 F+ = 70%; F+%[2]= 11,8%
K= 1; kan = 2 kan; 4 kp[3]
TRI 1/0 coartatif[4]; FS: 6/0 introverted RC% = 29,16;
6 A; 2 Ad; 1 (Ad); 1 H; 1 (H); 1 (Hd); 4 Hd; 1 Henf
$\rightarrow$ A% sans les (Ad) = 33.33% No respect of A/Ad ratio: 2Ad/6A
$\rightarrow$ H% (sans les (H), (Hd))= 25% No respect of H/Hd ratio: 4Hd/2H
IA%[5]= 33% (an = 3; sex =1; Hd = 4; no bl)
Popular = 0 (Popular) = 2;
Sex = 1; Anal Persp. = 3; Eq Choc = 1; Devit = 1; Ou = 1; Shock fragmentation = 1;
Abstract = 2; Eqe = 1; Rem int = 1; Crit obj = 1; Defect[6] = 2; Contam = 2; Confab = 1; Rem Neg = 1; Sym = 1; Anat = 3 Eyes Reference= 4; Phallic Reference = 5

---

1   F% means percentage of pure form responses (norm: 60%).
2   F+% means percentage of good form responses (norm: 65%).
3   K means Human Movement answers, kp means human part in movement, kan means animal in movement.
4   TRI means the ratio between human movement and answers generated by the color of the card. Coartatif means that one of these two types of answer is very scarce in the protocol.
5   IA% is an anxiety index related to self unity: it is the sum of Anatomic+ Sex+ Human part + Blood responses, divided by R, the total number answers (norm: 12%)
6   Defect means an answer with deteriorated content (similar to "MOR" content in American coding)

     Rorschachiana (2022), 43(1), 42–69

Table A1. Peter's Rorschach test following Nancy French Group coding

	Columns 1 2 3	Column 4
Card 1:		Eq. shock
Whoa… What does it mean here…?		
18" ^ 1. Carnival, wickedness, stern eyes…	1. D sup with the 2 superior white space	Paranoid projection
2.^ Wickedness, really, evil incarnate, and a smile like that, not vicious, just mean.	2. D inf	Paranoid projection
3. I'm angry when I see that… ^ 3. It's like a box that is closing, you know.	The malicious smile	Projective identification
Like that, it's fairly wide, it makes me say "huh"… Wow, you can spend a lot of time looking at that image.	Inferior middle of D medium with two white space area	Paranoid projection of mistrust and malicious intent
What's the point of all these tests I'm taking? To entrap me?		
2'33	3. Inferior middle of D medium	3. D F- Obj
This is giving me a headache…		
Card 2:		
4'?^		Criticism of the object
4. But there's no expression, no eyes, no mouth, no nose… an expression, isn't that something that can be read on someone's face?	4. Whole card and the white space area Face: Just like at a carnival, as I said, a mask	r4. W/S F- Hd/ Eyes	Projection of mistrust
5.^ And there, it looks like a penis which is going to penetrate a man. Ah, there I can perceive a sort of face there…You know, when you put on a hat.	5. D2 + D4	Obj Int Rem 5. D kp Sex/H	Raw projection of anal sexuality
That male organ, yuck		Crit Obj
[makes a face]		Anal.
1'47		Persp.Homosexual fantasy projection +++
		Anal regression+
Card 3:		Shock K
There are studies that are being done to….	6. D7	6. D F- (Hd)/Obj	paranoid projection
34"		Fragmentation projection
6.^ There, it looks like a skull with glasses, right there.		Defect
7.^ It looks like women's underwear… And there, it seems, a taking of control with respect to the skull… Like absolute evil with, uh… [shows the takeover with his hands].	7. Great white space around the central red details	7. D/S F- Cg/	–Confab Delusional paranoid projection Contam
It feels like we can't escape from an enclosed space … I don't see how any of this is useful for you…	This thing, it's paradoxical.	Abstract	Paranoid projection of confinement and mistrust
3'18"		
8. v Perhaps an animal like this, a sort of deer with antlers.	8. Antler picks D5	8. D F-A Phall. Ref	
9. v It looks like a small dog, too, with a small dog's head. 4'11	9. Dog (Dd33): there, the mussel the gaze, for the dog it doesn't go all the way to the top of the drawing	9. Dd F- Ad	

(Continued on next page)

Table A1. (continued)

Card 4: [Takes the card and looks at it with great astonishment] ^"10. An animal... A rooster with a very red neck.40" 1'19" I don't like it.	10. Whole card induced by D3 But there's no comb. It also looks like we are seeing it from behind. Additional response: Or someone who imposes himself, who falls, who sits down, plop. (Whole) W M- H Anal Perspective	10. DW F- A Phall ref Eq. shock Denial of reality (see reference to the color red) Anal Persp. Confab →Defect Criticism of the object
Card 5: ^ I can't make anything out... 11. An animal, a man who opens his wings, an animal with large... uh...not antennae, but, ah, yes... Oh, I don't know... Oh, shit... ^12. There I would say an animal as seen from behind; there are the back of the wings; from behind we can't see the eyes or anything; we only see it from behind and there is symmetry to its wings... 2'55	11. Here "antennae" D6 Whole card 12. Whole card	11. W- FM A/H Phal ref / Phallic reference/ Neg. Rem Telescoping H / A 12. W- F- ASym Loss of identity, no stability of identity, confusion of genders and species. Anal Perspect (Pop) Anal regression
Card 6: Whoa...5" ^13. An animal taking flight, a big animal, a giant, a giant. You see, people laughing, I feel they are making fun of me.^ 14. A big cat, a big head of a cat, a cat that has been run over... 15.^ And there we can see lungs there...What could it be... Not easy... 2'22	13. Whole card Ah, no, it was on the other one where there was the cat. 14. A cat does not have a face like that. Ah, yes, yes, with the whiskers there. [About people in another locale] Whole card 15. Dd32 (lungs)	13. W- FM- A/H Impermanence of the object → Phallic ref. 14. W- F- Ad Paranoid projection of persecution Defect Fragmentation projection 15. Dd F-An
Card 7: 13"^16. It looks like a fat woman's underwear. 17. ^ Ah, there are two tiny people, a baby with a tail, no, not a baby, I don't know, a sort of child, the sweet face of a child, a little girl. 1'36"	16. Whole card 17. Sweet face: D1 It's there at the top.	16. W- F- Cg 17. D F+ Hchild/ Hd child Phall. Ref Regression

(Continued on next page)

Table A1. (Continued)

Card 8:			
Whoa...			
10"^18. And that looks like a human body.	18. Whole card A human body that's been cut open	18. W- F- An →Defect	Fragmentation projection Repression attempt
With plastic surgery or something like that.			
19. ^ There, it looks like a small rat or a mouse, a fox.	19. D1	19. D F+A(Pop)	
20. ^ Here, it looks like vertebrae, right here	20. D3	20. D F- An	Projection of Fragmentation Contam
^21. It looks like a human stare or a tiger who is watching you and who's sulking.	21. Two white areas beside DS3 Stare: D white between the vertebrae	21. DdS kp Hd/Ad Or/Eyes/	Paranoid projection of mistrust and dangerousness Self-criticism
We need to focus, but it's not easy. I'm not a magician.			
2'20			
Card 9:			
There, it is difficult; perhaps there, but no...There, that one doesn't say anything...			
45"			
22. ^ Ah, yes, perhaps a nose with eyes perhaps. A snout, I would say, a snout of a pig.	22. DS1 (and white space) Snout D lat green white eyes	22. DS F- Ad Eyes 23. D M- H	Eq. shock Criticism of the object Paranoid projection
^ And not a very nice one at that...There, I would say that what is in green looks like	(in the green) D1+ space inside		
23. ^ a human being, staring off into space...	23. D1		
2'34			
Card 10:			
(Pursed lips, thinking...)			
1'27"			
^ Too complicated, tons of different things...			Shock M
24. Small demons, things...It's tough...	24. D1 (blue) (yellow) D2	24. D F- H	Fragmentation anxiety++ Paranoid projection of external danger
2'05"			

Table A2. R-PAS code sequence

R-PAS Code Sequence

C-ID: PETER - P-ID: 323 - Age: 37 - Gender: Male - Education: 16

Cd	#	Or	Loc	Loc #	SR	SI	Content	Sy	Vg	2	FQ	P	Determinants	Cognitive	Thematic	HR	ODL	R-Opt
I	1		Dd	99	SR	SI	(Hd)				o		Mp		ABS,AGM,AGC	PH	ODL	(RP)
	2		Dd	24			NC				-		ma					
II	3		W		SR	SI	(Hd)				o		F			GH		
III	4		Dd	99			Hd,Sx	Sy			-		Ma	FAB1	MAP	PH		
	5		D	7			An,NC	Sy			-		F					
	6		Dd	24			Cg,Sx	Sy			-		ma	DR2,FAB2	ABS,AGC,MAP			
	7	v	D	5			A				-		F					
	8	v	Dd	33			Ad				-		FMp					
IV	9		W				A				-		F					
V	10		W				H,A				o		Mp	DR2,FAB1		PH		
	11		W				A				o		F					
VI	12		W				A				u		FMa	DR2	MAP			
	13		W				A				o		F		MOR,MAP			
	14		Dd	32			An				u		F					
VII	15		W				Cg,Sx	Sy		2	-	P	F	FAB1			ODL	
	16		D	1			Hd				o		F	DV1		PH		
VIII	17		W				Hd				-	P	F	DR1	MAP	PH		
	18		D	1			A				o		F					
	19		D	3			An				o		F					
	20		Dd	99	SR		Hd,Ad				-		Mp,FMp		AGC	PH		
IX	21		D	1		SI	Ad				o		F				ODL	
	22		D	1			Hd				o		Mp			PH		
X	23		D	1,2			(H)				-		F		AGC	PH		

Table A3. R-PAS Protocol Level Counts & Calculation

R-PAS Protocol Level Counts & Calculations

C-ID: PETER P-ID: 323 Age: 37 Gender: Male Education: 16

Section	Counts		Counts		Calculations	
Responses & Administration	R = 23	R8910 = 7	Pr = 0	Pu = 0	R8910% = 30%	
	CT = 2					
Location	W = 8	D = 8	Dd = 7	WD = 16	W% = 35%	Dd% = 30%
Space	SR = 3	SI = 3	AnyS = 4			
Content	H = 1	An = 3	(H) = 1	Art = 0	SumH = 9	
	Hd = 5	Ay = 0	(Hd) = 2	Bl = 0	NPH = 8	
	A = 7	Cg = 2	(A) = 0	Ex = 0	NPH/SumH = 89%	
	Ad = 3	Fi = 0	(Ad) = 0	Sx = 3		
		NC = 2				
Object Qualities						
Synthesis	Sy = 4				Sy% = 17%	
Vagueness	Vg = 0				Vg% = 0%	
Pair	2 = 1					
Form Quality and Popular	FQo = 10	WDo = 9			FQo% = 43%	
	FQu = 2	WDu = 1			FQu% = 9%	
	FQ- = 11	WD- = 6			FQ-% = 48%	
	FQn = 0	WDn = 0			WD-% = 38%	
	M- = 2	P = 2				

Section	Counts		Counts		Calculations	
Determinants	M = 5	FC = 0			WSumC = 0.0	
Blends:	FM = 3	CF = 0			SumC = 0	
Mp,FMp	m = 2	C = 0			(CF+C)/SumC = NA	
	C' = 0	Y = 0			MC = 5.0	
	T = 0	V = 0			M/MC = 100%	
	r = 0	FD = 0			YTVC' = 0	
		F = 14			mY = 2	
					F% = 61%	
	a = 4	p = 6			PPD = 5	
	Ma = 1	Mp = 4			MC - PPD = 0.0	
	Blend = 1	CBlend = 0			p/(a+p) = 60%	
					Mp/(Ma+Mp) = 80%	
					Blend% = 4%	
Cognitive Codes	DV1 (1) = 1	DV2 (2) = 0			WSumCog = 41	
	INC1 (2) = 0	INC2 (4) = 0			SevCog = 4	
	DR1 (3) = 1	DR2 (6) = 3			Lev2Cog = 4	
	FAB1 (4) = 3	FAB2 (7) = 1				
	PEC (5) = 0	CON (7) = 0				
Thematic Codes	ABS = 2	PER = 0			MAHP = 5	
	COP = 0	MAH = 0			MAP/MAHP = 100%	
	AGM = 0	AGC = 4			GPHR = 9	
	MOR = 1	MAP = 5			PHR/GPHR = 89%	
	ODL = 3				ODL% = 13%	
	GHR = 1	PHR = 8				
Other Calculations	IntCont = 4	TP-Comp = 5.1	V-Comp = 4.9	SC-Comp = 5.2	Complexity = 58	
	CritCont% = 35%				LSO = 27	
	EII-3 = 4.0				Cont = 21	
					Det = 10	

Counts and Calculations in Bold Font are on the Summary Scores and Profiles Pages

Table A4. R-PAS Summary Score and Profiles – Page 1

R-PAS Summary Scores and Profiles – Page 1

C-ID: PETER   P-ID: 323   Age: 37   Gender: Male   Education: 16

Domain/Variables	Raw Scores	Raw %ile	Raw SS	Cplx. Adj. %ile	Cplx. Adj. SS	Standard Score Profile R-Optimized										Abbr.
						60	70	80	90	100	110	120	130	140	
Admin. Behaviors and Obs.															
Pr	0	24	89						90						Pr
Pu	0	40	96						96						Pu
CT (Card Turning)	2	44	98						98						CT
Engagement and Cog. Processing						60	70	80	90	100	110	120	130	140	
Complexity	58	25	90						90						Cmplx
R (Responses)	23	46	99	56	102				99						R
F% [Lambda=1.56] (Simplicity)	61%	86	116	78	110					116					F%
Blend	1	14	84	31	92		84								Bln
Sy	4	27	91	50	100				91						Sy
MC	5.0	31	92	47	99				92						MC
MC - PPD	0.0	68	107	67	107						107				MC-PPD
M	5	72	109	77	111						109				M
M/MC [5/5.0]	100%	99	135	99	142									135	M Prp
(CF+C)/SumC [0/0]	NA														CFC Prp
Perception and Thinking Problems						60	70	80	90	100	110	120	130	140	
EII-3	4.0	>99	143	>99	143									143	EII
TP-Comp (Thought & Percept. Com...)	5.1	99	142	99	142									142	TP-C
WSumCog	41	>99	142	>99	144									142	WCog
SevCog	4	99	138	99	138									138	Sev
FQ-%	48%	>99	143	>99	143									143	FQ-%
WD-%	38%	>99	143	>99	143									143	WD-%
FQo%	43%	11	82	5	75		82								FQo%
P	2	4	73	8	78	73									P
Stress and Distress						60	70	80	90	100	110	120	130	140	
YTVC'	0	3	73	11	81	73									YTVC'
m	2	66	106	67	107						106				m
Y	0	17	85	24	88		85								Y
MOR	1	51	100	55	102					100					MOR
SC-Comp (Suicide Concern Comp.)	5.2	69	108	74	110						108				SC-C
Self and Other Representation						60	70	80	90	100	110	120	130	140	
ODL%	13%	66	106	70	108						106				ODL%
SR (Space Reversal)	3	92	122	92	122							122			SR
MAP/MAHP [5/5]	100%	94	123	92	122							123			MAP Prp
PHR/GPHR [8/9]	89%	99	133	99	133									133	PHR Prp
M-	2	94	123	94	123							123			M-
AGC	4	70	108	71	109						108				AGC
H	1	21	88	29	91			88							H
COP	0	21	88	39	96			88							COP
MAH	0	26	90	26	90				90						MAH

© 2010-2018 R-PAS

Original Article

Color and Affect

A Long, Never-Ending History

Anna Elisa de Villemor-Amaral[1] and Latife Yazigi[2]

[1]Graduate Program of Psychology, São Francisco University, Campinas, Brazil
[2]Department of Psychiatry, Federal University of São Paulo, Brazil

Abstract: This work arose from an interest in seeking the origins, in the field of psychological assessment, of knowledge on the relationship between color and affect. This relationship in psychological assessment has existed since Herman Rorschach published his book *Psychodiagnostics*. In 1967 Beck stated that it was not Rorschach who discovered the relationship between color and affectivity, recognizing that there was evidence that this relationship had been accepted since the early days of civilization. In the 1940s, studies on painting and personality and on the artistic production of psychotic patients began to appear more prominently and culminated in Buck's work, with his suggestion for inclusion of colors in the HTP test. In the 1950s, Pfister and Lücher published their color tests, with some theoretical considerations about the cultural and physiological aspects related to the symbolic interpretation of colors. Neuroscience can now be used to better understand how color perception and processing work in the brain, although the connection between color and affect in this field needs to be explored more. Studies in different areas such as physics, anthropology, ethology, and sociology suggest that a combination of factors related to the qualities of the light stimulus and its perception are also associated with the colors in nature and their symbolism that lead to the affective connotations of colors.

Keywords: emotions, projective techniques, psychological assessment

This article arose out of an interest in verifying the origin of the relationship between color and affectivity in the field of psychological assessment. The idea that responses to colored stimuli reveal personality characteristics related to affectivity has been part of the field of psychological assessment since Hermann Rorschach published his book *Psychodiagnostics* in 1921[1]. In the chapter "The Affectivity. The Personality" Rorschach explained (1921/1981):

---

[1]   The authors are aware that a new version of Hermann Rorschach's book *Psychodiagnostics* has been recently released and of its new features (see Aschieri, 2022, in this issue). However, since the present paper was prepared before publication of the book, the references in the text are based on the English translation published in 1981.

Rorschachiana (2022), 43(1), 70–88
https://doi.org/10.1027/1192-5604/a000156

We gather together under the term "Affectivity" the emotions, the affects, the feelings of pleasure and displeasure. The test gives orientation as to the affective status of the subject. It gives information as to the stability or instability, strength or weakness of the feelings, the intensivity or extensivity of the affective reaction, the control of lack of control over the reactions, the suppression or freedom of reaction. (pp. 98–99)

Rorschach considered that the number of color responses was a good measure of affective lability, and the number of pure color responses (C) indicated the amount of affective lability, which the subject actually shows. He stated:

It has been found empirically that the influence of colors in perceiving the figures may be taken to represent the extent of emotional excitability and actual excitement; the basis for this deduction is, however, quite insufficient to satisfy the demands of scientific logic. (p. 98)

After discussing the role of color in the perceptions, he concluded:

It has long been realized that there must exist a remarkably close relationship between color and affectivity. The gloomy person is one to whom everything looks "black", while the cheerful person is said to see everything through rose-colored glasses. (p. 99)

As far back as it is possible to examine Rorschach's ideas prior to this date, there was no mention of the use of an association between color and affectivity to identify personality characteristics[2]. Beck (1967) acknowledged that Rorschach was not the first to establish the connection between color and affect, since this link already existed "at the dawn of civilization" (p. 130), and that Rorschach used this idea that was deeply entrenched in human belief, without worrying about conducting studies to confirm it. It was so obvious that he simply took it for granted.

Ellenberger (1954) deduced from a coherent sequence of ideas the pathway that H. Rorschach most likely followed in his work to reach the relation between color responses and extroversion and movement responses and introversion. In *Psychodiagnostics*, Rorschach (1921/1981) presented the results of his trials involving the perception of inkblots, in both psychiatric patients and nonclinical people. The relationship between color and affect was empirically based on his observation of

[2] Editor note: Rita Signer, one of the coauthors of the 2021 version of *Psychodiagnostics* (Rorschach, 1921/2021), provides more information on the early articulations of Hermann Rorschach views on the Rorschach Test and color.

people's reactions to the various types of stimuli, whether colored or not. In the very first pages of his book, he presented data from his observations of the quantity and quality of color responses in people diagnosed with epilepsy and compared the results with those of patients diagnosed with depression, who presented few color responses.

Considering this line of thinking, Silberstein (2011) recounted that Rorschach identified the movement determinant in schizophrenia-like psychoses, the form determinant in patients with severe depression, and the color determinant as a characteristic of mania, a type of "affective psychosis." He concluded, "Starting from this moment, but not only for this reason, color is found in the theory in relation to affect" (p. 93).

Recently, Searls (2017) remarked that Rorschach started to give Color responses a deeper psychological meaning. "None of his earlier work had paid color much attention of any kind" (p. 134). He explains that Rorschach used the word *affect* to mean emotional reactions, either feelings or expressions of feeling. "A person's 'affectivity' was their mode of feeling, how they were 'affected' by things" (p. 134). He mentioned Rorschach's insights, finding that individuals with stable affect, calm reactions, insensitivity, or depression presented few or no color responses, and individuals with labile or volatile affect, with strong reactions, or oversensitivity presented many color responses. He commented, "Again, Rorschach fails to ground this insight in any theory, beyond the nearly universal folk wisdom that we react emotionally to color. He claimed only that he had noticed the correlation in practice" (p. 135).

Therefore, the relationship between color and affect was established in the field of psychological assessment for the first time, without any theoretical formulation on the matter. Rorschach (1921/1981) drew attention to the differences in the responses in which form plays a more or less important role in the person's associative process and he established the importance of carefully determining which aspect of the stimulus most influenced the response, the form or the color. Then, he created an experiment to observe the extent to which a person's answers to the test were guided by color or by form through the presentation of pictures of animals where the shape and color were not congruent, such as a cat colored as a frog or a squirrel colored as a cockerel. In these "ambiguous" figures, some people were more influenced by the color when identifying a frog or a cockerel, while others were influenced by the form when identifying a cat or a squirrel.

The introversion–extroversion polarity became an axis of personality that led to the creation of the type of experience, which for Ellenberger (1954) was the central aspect of *Psychodiagnostics*. According to Ellenberger (1954), Rorschach probably received suggestions about color from his friend Fankhauser, who had imagined a "sphere of emotions" giving a graphic representation of every possible nuance of emotion in a three-dimensional frame; in which the emotions were considered as the combination of three pairs of the three antagonistic emotions. It was an imitation of the "sphere of colors" of Wundt, which gives a graphic representation of the three complementary colors (p. 202). This affective polyhedron (*Affektkörper*) based on Wundt's color sphere (*Farbenkugel*) was presented in his *Principles of Physiological Psychology* (1910), being a three-dimensional graphic representation of a theory of emotions.

In his introversion–extroversion typology, Rorschach (1921/1981) refers to them as two universal psychological functions, with both being effective and active, emphasizing that they are not two constitutional types that exclude each other. For Rorschach (1921/1981) the two functions are necessary both for the individual and for mankind. He stated that: "Introversives are cultured, extratensives are civilized" (p. 110), and that: "Culture always grows out of introversion; civilization is an extratensive adaptation and usage, but is not, in itself, culture" (p. 113). Quoting Ellenberger (1954): "Introversion will be the basis of culture and extroversion will be the basis of civilization" (p. 103).

Shapiro (1977) recognized that the Rorschach problem of the interpretative meaning of color response had not been a subject of much debate among clinical Rorschach workers. Some were convinced of the linkage but not of the rationale by simply assuming some sort of given intrinsic affective value of color. Others assumed the existence of culturally established, highly charged, and affective associations with colors.

Schachtel (1966) remarked that the perception of color, if it is not accompanied by, and integrated with, the perception of form, typically occurs with a passive, more autocentric perceptual attitude. "Color and light impinge on the eye, which does not have to seek them out attentively but *reacts* to their impact. Color seizes the eye, but the eye grasps form" (p. 160). For this author there are two common characteristics of color experience and affective experience: the *passivity* of the subject and the *immediacy* of the subject–object relationship. Both refer to the *striking* character of color. Therefore, color perception is essentially passive and this process accounts for the main attributes of extratensive individuals in Rorschach's original formulation.

Also Bash (1984) expressed concern about the theoretical foundation of the Rorschach method. He stated that:

> There is undoubtedly a lack of theoretical foundation on the meaning of color responses, which are viewed as characteristic of the individual's affectivity. This is not the case with kinesthesias, or movement responses, which have been shown to be related to the inner world of the individual. The simple dualistic explanation that identifies color as the objective aspect and the

affect as the subjective aspect of an event is not sustainable. Objectively there are no colors, but only light waves of certain frequencies. Moreover, the perception of color is fairly regularly accompanied by affect, but not the converse. (p. 847)

Bash (1984) employed Köhler's (1929) and Metzger's (1954) notions of "properties of organized wholes" to examine the Rorschach determinants. According to his concepts: (a) *Essence* or physiognomic characteristics is what most easily arouses affect. Pure colors, being pure essence, account for the chromatic determinant. (b) *Structure* reveals itself in form, accounting for the form determinant. (c) *Quality,* the nature, condition or property of a thing, is best seen in shading, whereby the use of this determinant indicates the prevailing quality of mood. (d) *Movement* is determined by structure, but also by the capacity for dynamic resonance and human intimacy.

Regarding the symbolic meaning of certain colors, Ellenberger (1954) said that Fankhauser was the first to imagine a system of analogies between colors and the emotional life. It seems likely that he inspired Rorschach's idea of connecting color perception and affectivity: red with impulsivity and blue with self-control. Rorschach, however, did not make this acknowledgment and he could also have used his own clinical observations or even common sense (Ellenberger, 1954).

From this point of view, Rorschach (1921/1981) also drew attention to the use of the colors black, white, and gray and the importance of distinguishing them from other color responses. He also mentioned the symbolic connotations of black, pink, and colorful military uniforms (p. 99). He referred to the differences between people, indicating that a preference for blue and green figures was typical of people who control their emotions (p. 35), although this type of consideration is not part of the method he developed.

Specific Colors, Specific Meanings

It is important to remember that it was Newton, in the 18th century, who discovered that colors are a phenomenon of light and paved the way for a better understanding of the relationships between color and affects. Knowing Newton's theory, Goethe (1810) challenged his theory; however, he was more interested in describing his many experiments on the emotional effect that colors, considering them as a phenomenon of light, have on people. Concerning the history that came later, Maier et al. (2009) reported that it was Jonas Cohn who in 1894, in Wundt's laboratory, performed the first study on color preference and personality. Later, Ostwald (1931, cited by Eysenck, 1941) described, together with considerations about physical and chemical aspects of colors, the experiments he performed based on psychological aspects. Eysenck (1941) himself states the importance for psychology of studies on the effects of colors.

Decades later, Jacobs and Hustmeyer (1974) conducted experiments to determine the effects of primary colors on manifestations of the autonomic nervous system, namely, galvanic skin response (GSR), heart rate, and respiration. He confirmed the positive findings of various predecessors, quoting Wilson and Gerard's results (Wilson & Gerard, 1954, as cited by Jacobs & Hustmeyer, 1974), who discovered, through physiological measures, such as heart rate, GSR, eye blinking, blood pressure, and changes in EEG, the extent to which the color red is more stimulating than the color green. The authors also mentioned the work of Nourse and Welch (1971, as cited by Jacobs & Hustmeyer, 1974), who found that the color violet is more stimulating than the color green, observing that the composition of the color violet they used had a higher percentage of red, corroborating Wilson and Gerard's findings.

Concerning psychological assessment, it was in the 1940s that studies on painting and personality and on the artistic creation of psychotic patients became more prominent, culminating in the work of Buck, in 1948, who suggested to include colors in the House–Tree–Person (HTP) test (Buck, 1948/2003). However, it was only in 1958 that Hammer (1958) extended Buck's ideas. He considered that color drawings made in crayon reveal deeper layers of the personality and express the subject's reactions to and tolerance of emotional stimuli, in the same way as the Rorschach method.

In the 1950s, Birren (1950) presented his historical study in which he states that since ancient times, colors were used by druids and, during the Middle Ages, by alchemists, as a treatment for physical diseases. He notes that paganism, given its love of nature, valued colors, whereas other religions valued the symbolic aspects of colors related to the gods and their powers. According to the author, the underlying significance of these notions is the fact that color is a luminous phenomenon, with light, from the sun, being essential for life in all its forms.

Also in the 1950s, Pfister developed his Color Pyramid Test, based on the choice of 10 colors and 24 hues to complete three bi-dimensional pyramid shapes. However, he did not present any further theoretical considerations on the connection between color and personality trends (Villemor-Amaral, 2014). Pfister (cited by Schaie & Heiss, 1964) empirically observed the relationship between colors and certain affective states from his experience as a choreographer and scenographer, based on the effects of colors on audience reactions during performances. To some extent, this can be considered an experiment that, just like for Rorschach, led to a discovery that was yet to be supported by theory.

Not long afterwards, Lücher (1974) published his Color Test. It is in this book that we find, for the first time in the context of psychological assessment, some theoretical considerations on the cultural and physiological aspects related to the interpretation of colors. The author stated that:

> In the beginning, man's life was dictated by two factors that were beyond his control: night and day, darkness and light. Night brought about an environment in which action had to cease, so man repaired to his cave, wrapped himself with his furs and went to sleep. Or he climbed a tree and made himself as comfortable as he could while awaiting the coming of dawn. (p. 15)

He also clarified that, from the standpoint of physiology, experiments had already been conducted that demonstrated the stimulating effects of the color red on the autonomic nervous system, increasing blood pressure and speeding up both the respiration rate and heartbeat. The reverse effect was produced by pure blue.

Contributions From Neurosciences

The neurosciences provided contributions on how color perception is processed in the brain and whether this processing confirms the relationship between the perception of color stimuli and affect. In the field of hemispheric brain specialization, Levy and Trevarthen (1981) described their investigation on the lateralization of brain functions related to the perception of colors. They demonstrated that the capacity to name colors depends on the integrity of the visual fields of the left hemisphere while the capacity to discriminate colors depends on the integrity of the visual fields of the right hemisphere. This is because the strategies of the left hemisphere rely on language or language-related functions, whereas the functions of the right hemisphere depend on image constructions closely representing the sensory experience. Both hemispheres showed good performance in relation to memory for colors of objects; however, the right hemisphere performed better than the left.

Levy and Trevarthen (1981) pointed out that various studies reveal that the right hemisphere is superior for color discrimination when the colors are difficult to name or describe, while equality between the two hemispheres was found when the colors come from an easily nameable set. This nameable–non-nameable distinction, say the authors, is similar to that pertaining to shapes. Investigations of people without neurological problems support the conclusion that both hemispheres play an important role in color perception and naming. As such, discrimination and memory for nameable stimuli or stimuli that are easy to describe may be equal for the two hemispheres, although through different cognitive operations.

Ornstein (1975/1984), equated the left hemisphere of the brain with a rational and logical way of Western thinking, as in Freud's conscious; and the right hemisphere with an intuitive and mystic Eastern way of thinking, as in Freud's unconscious. Schore (2002) corroborated Ornstein's claim that the right hemisphere is the neurological substrate of Freud's unconscious, and he added that the right hemisphere has a strong connection to the limbic system and subcortical regions dominant in processing emotion, so that highly affective experiences predominantly activate the right hemisphere, more specifically the subcortical regions.

These studies show to what extent the sensory grasp of stimuli, regardless of the action of the cognitive functions, is processed by the right hemisphere, this also being where the records of the more primary emotional experiences lie, which contributes toward neurologically demonstrating the correlation between affect and color response.

Concerning the lateralization, Bash (1984) conducted an experiment with a two-channel tachistoscope in which the Rorschach inkblots were presented unilaterally. They described the differences found for several response coding variables. The authors reported that, with an exposure of 50 ms, "[...] we did find significantly more FC and FC+ responses in the right hemisphere, and at 150 ms a trend for CF responses from the same side, however, the hypothesized difference between Sum FC on the left hemisphere and Sum (CF+C) on the right hemisphere was not confirmed" (Bash et al., 1984, p. 4). The authors stated that the right hemisphere, as a result, is not more "colorful," or consequently more emotional than the left, when considering the dominance of form as criteria.

In another paper, Regard and Landis (1988) commented on the results of the previously mentioned study:

> 57% of the interpretations differed when the same inkblot was presented to the left visual field or to the right visual field, for example: "dark evil man with big feet" (right hemisphere) or "frog" (left hemisphere). Twenty-seven percent of the responses were similar but differently verbalized, for example: "dark evil man with big feet" or "black giant". Only 16% of the responses were completely identical in both visual fields. A trend analysis revealed that most subjects differed significantly in their responses determined by form, color or movement according to right or left visual field stimulation. (p. 252)

In conclusion, the authors stated that the interpretations of inkblots differ according to the hemisphere stimulated and they reflect hemispheric differences in affective-visual processing. Since the differences were primarily in the way the two hemispheres dealt with the emotional stimulus in the inkblots, shape recognition differed little.

Yazigi (1995), in her investigation of patients undergoing neurosurgery for the treatment of intractable epilepsy, who were studied from a psychological viewpoint using the Rorschach, observed that the intergroup study confirmed the findings of the concepts regarding the lateralization of the Rorschach components. The patients with right temporal epilepsy who had a right temporal lobectomy showed bias toward affective susceptibility and responsiveness as well as emotional reactions such as dysphoria, anxiety, and anguish.

According to the observations on the relation between brain functioning and Freud's theory of affect, Schore (2002) demonstrated the predominance of the right hemisphere in nonverbal communication between mother and infant, and how situations of conflict in the early stages of life produce disruptions in the functioning of this hemisphere that will express themselves in emotional difficulties that appear throughout life.

Finn (2012) drew on Schore to show that in psychological assessment processes, the combination of self-report tests and projective tests demonstrates that the response to each of these types of test expresses different brain functioning. Scales depend more on the activation of the left hemisphere, whereas in the responses to projective tests the right hemisphere plays a more significant role, particularly when the responses have more affect. These data corroborate the idea that the emotions are more intense when the right hemisphere is activated, as stated by Regard and Landis (1988) in their previously cited experiments.

According to Hurlbert and Ling (2017), the eye and the brain contribute significant processing power to seeing in color, since color is fundamentally a contextual phenomenon, which depends on the sensory information that has come previously, and which emanates simultaneously from the surroundings. Complex neuronal circuits participate in the decoding of information from the light beam that is associated not only with the perception of shape and depth, but also with the expectations of the person who perceives it, through the memory records. This allows the person to recognize and give name and meaning to what is perceived, already at cortical levels. However, Gegenfurtner and Kiper (2003) stated that the processes that integrate color with these other visual attributes to form neural representations of objects, and the areas of the brain in which these processes occur, are still not fully understood. Zeki and Marini (1998) argued that humans are basically visual animals and that the best way to understand the functioning of the human brain would be to unveil the process of vision. Trying to understand how the brain sees the world, the authors showed that in addition to a primary visual reception center (V1), in the cerebral cortex, the function of which is to see and interpret what we see, there are several other areas implicated in visual perception, therefore establishing the principle of multiplicity in the visual system. They affirmed that the V4 area of the brain is responsible for the visual processing of color. There, neurons relate and compare the wavelengths reflected by an object with the wavelengths reflected by all other objects around it, performing a series of processing tasks. Later, Zeki and Bartels (1999) stated that in this area (V4) there are some cells that respond better to different colors. However, in their paper it is not clear whether they are talking about the importance of V4 for the reactivity to the wavelengths or for the recognition and naming of colors. Considering the data presented by Levy and Trevarthen (1981), as highlighted previously in this paper, it is possible that Zeki and Bartels (1999) was talking about recognition and naming, independent of hemispheres but both at cortical levels.

In the same direction, Ishibashi et al. (2017) sought to verify the impact of the chromatic stimulus on the different regions of the brain, during the administration of the Rorschach. They also identified a significant activation of the V4 brain area at the moment when the colored boards were presented. This was a thorough and in-depth study of the different reactions observed in the brain when comparing reactions to achromatic and chromatic cards. However, the focus of these authors was on the differences in the perception processes of the two types of stimuli – chromatic and achromatic – without attempting to address the relationships between color and affects.

Hartz (2019), in a literature review of color and emotion on the Rorschach, found various studies on the theme, since the research in the 1940s and 1950s on color shock, until the ones examining differences in the physiological activity [of the brain] when the color was the response determinant. He concludes that, "it's not clear that they [studies] have any bearing on the question of why color is linked to activating emotion or negative affect" (Hartz, 2019, p. 32).

Another perspective regarding color perception and affect came from some research into Parkinson's disease. Li et al. (2018) showed that patients with Parkinson's who had higher scores on the Beck II Depression Inventory (BDI-II) have more difficulty distinguishing colors. The authors concluded that more severe depressive symptoms are associated with worse color vision. One of the main reasons they found was the link between the impairment in color vision and low levels of dopamine that, among several physiological effects, produced a constriction of the pupil that reduced the perception of luminosity and brightness. Life is seen as less vibrant and stimulating in depression due to the interaction of physiological and psychological aspects, the latter arising from the association of vivid and bright colors with more excited or intense emotional states.

All these considerations help to demonstrate that color perception is related to emotions, both manifested with more significant activation of the right hemisphere. The naming of colors, like the recognition and naming of emotions, involves more cognitive processing predominantly associated with the left hemisphere. This idea can also be corroborated by the findings of Silva (2016), who demonstrated a reduction in the production of responses to colored cards among children. This suggested to the author that this reduction could result from the difficulty in responding, in an operatively correct way, due to the presence of color, which then serves as an inhibitor of the response in this age group. Therefore, an increase in responses to colored cards, starting in adolescence, would be justified by the acquisition, through cognitive development, of greater mastery of the perceptual operations involved in the response.

It should be noted that in the examples selected here from the neuroscience literature, concerning the perception of colors and their relationships with affects and emotions, the issue related to universally shared associations between certain colors and certain emotions was not addressed. Considering that different colors are created by different types of light waves, with their respective frequencies and lengths, it still does not seem totally clear how these differences impact neurologically and psychologically.

However, Elliot (2015) mentioned several works exploring the impact of color on emotions and psychological functions. One of them, investigating the relation between color and selective attention, found that red stimuli received an attentional advantage. Another study showed that blue light increased subjective alertness and performance in attention-based tasks. According to a literature review by Elliot (2015), studies on color and athletic performance have linked wearing red to better performance and perceived performance in sports competitions and tasks. Other studies showed that: Viewing red prior to a challenging cognitive task undermined performance; viewing red on oneself or others increased appraisals of aggressiveness and dominance; viewing red in achievement contexts increased caution and avoidance; viewing red on or near a female has been shown to enhance attraction in heterosexual males; blue in stores/logos increases quality and trustworthiness appraisals; and finally, citing only some of the studies compiled by Elliot (2015), red influenced food and beverage perception and consumption. More recent studies on the matter coincide with several aspects and corroborate the studies cited (see Chai et al., 2019; Hanada, 2018; Ikeda, 2020; Jonauskaite, Parraga, et al., 2020; Kawai et al., 2020).

Color and Culture

There is the possibility of exploring, in culture and in psychology, the origin of the ideas about how specific colors correspond to different qualities of emotions. These notions that the distinct impacts of colors are linked to distinct impacts of emotions have been entrenched in cultural manifestations since ancient times. Rorschach did not develop his ideas any further in this respect, while neither Lücher nor Pfister demonstrated this scientifically.

We can find in papers from other areas of knowledge, such as anthropology, sociology, and even linguistics, several studies that have sought to verify connections between certain colors and certain emotions; however, the results do not always point in the same direction (Villemor-Amaral, 2014), although there are considerable similarities among some of them. This is because the research varies widely concerning the type of color stimulation that is used in each experiment: whether it is printed, whether it is projected, whether it is named or not, and whether it is associated with words and objects. The various depths and infinite varieties of each tone also make it difficult to compare results. Nevertheless, in general it is possible to show that the emotional meaning of each basic color has been linked to the relationship between humans and nature since primitive times. Hurlbert and Ling (2007) speculated that women could discriminate red faster than men could due to their need to identify ripe fruit among the leaves. They also report that the perception of movement, by contrast, developed more in primitive men than in women due to men's need to identify prey when hunting. This finding is in line with the study on languages and color naming conducted by Berlin and Kay (1969), who discovered that in all languages, besides the words to designate light and dark that originated from the experience of day and night in nature, the first color that was given a name was red and the last was blue. They deduced that this marks the origin of language based on the needs of humans, indicating that red is linked to food (ripe fruit and the blood of slaughtered prey) whereas there is practically nothing in nature that serves as food that is blue, making the naming of this color less necessary in the origin of oral language.

It is possible to find a certain number of studies from the past decades that show the relationship between being exposed to some colors and typical emotional reactions, as Goethe aimed to do in the 19th century.

Jonauskaite, Abu-Akel et al. (2020) demonstrated, through an extensive and sophisticated methodology, that there are universal patterns in the associations between certain colors and certain affects and emotions. According to the authors, the origin of these associative patterns is anchored in long-standing concepts throughout human history, shared globally through similarities in language and in the environment. As an example of these universal associations, they mention black being associated with sadness, while love and anger are associated with red. The study also revealed some variations in these associations, which are geographically determined, leading to the conclusion that the greater the linguistic and geographical proximity, the greater the similarity in the associations between colors and affects.

Conclusion

We began this essay by investigating how, in the context of psychological assessment, color became a means of interpreting affective dynamics (in the Rorschach Test) and how each color became associated with specific emotions (Pfister and Lücher tests; graphic tests). The data indicate that the authors of the psychological assessment techniques based the considerations about emotions and color in their methods on accepted cultural facts and on their own clinical observations. Later studies in physics and then in the neurosciences, prompted by the advances in technologies for observing brain functioning, enabled progress on the understanding of the relation between color and emotion and, more recently, studies have shown the impact of biochemical factors on the perception of colors by producing changes in the ocular globe and pupil movements, such as the effects of dopamine. Meanwhile, studies from other areas of knowledge, such as the humanities and social sciences, have demonstrated the extent to which each color, with its intrinsic qualities, is associated with different emotions.

As a final point, it is important to emphasize that one of the fundamental problems when studying these issues is the fact that objectively colors are not in the objects; they are a phenomenon of light formed by waves of different lengths and frequencies. From the point of view of affect, what distinguishes so-called warm colors from cold colors is the fact that the former are more stimulating and the latter are more calming. Furthermore, in addition to the basic colors, there are infinite variations of tones and brightness, which makes the control of variables more difficult in research on the subject. The perspectives of physics, neuroscience, anthropology, ethology, and sociology have contributed to the understanding of the phenomenon of color and affect. There is a combination of factors regarding the quality of the light stimulus that is associated with the colors in nature and with the cultural symbolism of colors that lead to their affective connotations. The complexity evolved in this matter and the innumerous possible perspectives open several doors and show that psychological science still has a great deal to offer in a long never-ending history.

References

Aschieri, F. (2022). Hermann Rorschach's psychodiagnostics [Book review]. *Rorschachiana, 43*(1), 89–94. https://doi.org/10.1027/1192-5604/a000154
Bash, K. W. (1984). Whole properties: Determinants of determinants. *Perceptual and Motor Skills, 59*, 847–851.

Bash, K. W., Regard, N., & Landis, T. (1984, July). *Tachistoscopic Rorschach presentation to the several cerebral hemispheres* [Paper presentation]. XI International Rorschach Congress, Barcelona, Spain.

Beck, S. (1967). *Le test du Rorschach* [The Rorschach Test]. PUF.

Berlin, B., & Kay, P. (1969). *Basic color terms. Their universality and evolution*. University of California Press.

Birren, F. (1950). *Color psychology and color therapy. A factual study of the influence of color on human life*. University Books.

Buck, J. N. (1948/2003). *Casa, Arvore e Pessoa. HTP. Manual e Guia de Interpretação*. Vetor.

Chai, M. T., Amin, H. U., Izhar, L. I., Saad, M. N. M., Rahman, M. A., Malik, A. S., & Tang, T. B. (2019). Exploring EEG effective connectivity network in estimating influence of color on emotion and memory. *Frontiers in Neuroinformatics, 13*, Article 66. https://doi.org/10.3389/fninf.2019.00066

Ellenberger, H. (1954). The life and work of Hermann Rorschach. *Bulletin of the Menninger Clinic, 18*(5), 173–219.

Elliot, A. J. (2015). Color and psychological functioning: A review of theoretical and empirical work. *Frontiers in Psychology, 6*, Article 368. https://doi.org/10.3389/fpsyg.2015.00368

Eysenck, H. J. (1941). A critical and experimental study of colour preferences. *The American Journal of Psychology, 54*(3), 385–394. https://doi.org/10.2307/1417683

Finn, E. S. (2012). Implications of recent research in neurobiology for psychological assessment. *Journal of Personality Assessment, 94*(5), 440–449.

Gegenfurtner, K. R., & Kiper, D. C. (2003). Color vision. *Annual Review of Neuroscience, 26*, 181–206. https://doi.org/10.1146/annurev.neuro.26.041002.131116

Hammer, E. F. (1958). *The clinical application of projective drawings*. Charles C. Thomas.

Hanada, M. (2018). Correspondence analysis of color-emotion associations. *Color Research and Application, 43*(2), 224–237. https://doi.org/10.1002/col.22171

Hartz, A. (2019). *Embodied associations beyond the Rorschach: Color, emotion, and personality* [Doctoral dissertation]. Long Island University, The Brooklyn Center.

Hurlbert, A. C., & Ling, Y. (2007). Biological components of sex differences in color preference. *Current Biology, 17*(16), 623–625. https://doi.org/10.1016/j.cub.2007.06.022

Hurlbert, A. C., & Ling, Y. (2017). Understanding colour perception and preference. In J. Best (Ed.), *Colour design: Theories and applications* (pp. 169–192). Elsevier.

Ikeda, S. (2020). Influence of color on emotion recognition is not bidirectional: An investigation of the association between color and emotion using a stroop-like task. *Psychological Reports, 123*(4), 1226–1239. https://doi.org/10.1177/0033294119850480

Ishibashi, M., Uchiumi, C., Jung, M., Aizawa, N., Makita, K., Nakamura, Y., & Saito, D. N. (2017). Differences in brain hemodynamics in response to achromatic and chromatic cards of the Rorschach. A fMRI study. *Rorschachiana, 37*(1), 41–57. https://doi.org/10.1027/1192-5604/a000076

Jacobs, K. W., & Hustmeyer, F. E. Jr. (1974). Effects of four psychological primary colors on GSR, heart rate, and respiration rate. *Perceptual and Motor Skills, 38*, 736–766.

Jonauskaite, D., Abu-Akel, A., Dael, N., Oberfeld, D., Abdel-Khalek, A. M., Al-Rasheed, A. S., Antonietti, J. P., Bogushevskaya, V., Chamseddine, A., Chkonia, E., Corona, V., Fonseca-Pedrero, E., Griber, Y. A., Grimshaw, G., Hasan, A. A., Havelka, J., Hirnstein, M., Karlsson, B. S. A., ... Mohr, C. (2020). Universal patterns in color-emotion associations are further shaped by linguistic and geographic proximity. *Psychological Science, 31*(10), 1245–1260.

Jonauskaite, D., Parraga, C. A., Quiblier, M., & Mohr, C. (2020). Feeling blue or seeing red? Similar patterns of emotion associations with colour patches and colour terms. *i-Perception, 11*(1), 1–24. https://doi.org/101177/2041669520902484

Kawai, C., Lukács, G., & Ansorge, U. (2020). Polarities influence implicit associations between colour and emotion. *Acta Psychologica, 209*, Article 103143. https://doi.org/10.1016/j.actpsy.2020.103143

Köhler, W. (1929). *Gestalt psychology*. Liveright.

Levy, J., & Trevarthen, C. (1981). Color-matching, color-naming and color-memory in split-brain patients. *Neuropsychologia, 4*, 523–541.

Li, D. K., Liu, F. T., Chen, K., Bu, L. L., Yang, K., Chen, C., Liu, Z. Y., Tang, Y. L., Zhao, J., Sun, Y. M., Wang, J., & Wu, J. J. (2018). Depressive symptoms are associated with color vision but not olfactory function in patients with Parkinson's disease. *The Journal of Neuropsychiatry and Clinical Neurosciences, 30*(2), 122–129. https://doi.org/10.1176/appi.neuropsych.17030063

Lücher, M. (1974). *Test de los colores* [Color test]. Paidós.

Maier, M. A., Barchfeld, P., Elliot, A. J., & Pekrun, R. (2009). Context specificity of implicit preferences: The case of human preference for red. *Emotion, 9*(5), 734–738.

Metzger, W. (1954). *Psychologie* [Psychology]. Steinkopf.

Ornstein, R. E. (1975/1984). *The psychology of consciousness*. Penguin Books.

Regard, M., & Landis, T. (1988). Beauty may differ in each half of the eye of the beholder. In I. Rentschler, B. Herzberger, & D. Esptein (Eds.), *Beauty and the brain: Biological aspects of aesthetics* (pp. 243–256). Birkhauser.

Rorschach, H. (1981). *Psychodiagnostics: A diagnostic test based on perception*. Hans Huber. (Original work published 1921)

Rorschach, H. (2021). *Hermann Rorschach's psychodiagnostics: Newly translated and annotated 100th anniversary edition* (P. J. Keddy, R. Signer, P. Erdberg, & A. Schneider-Stocking, Eds. & Trans.). Hogrefe Publishing. (Original work published 1921)

Schachtel, E. G. (1966). *Experiential foundations of Rorschach's test*. Basic Books.

Schaie, W., & Heiss, R. (1964). *Color and personality: A manual for the color pyramid test*. Hans Huber.

Schore, A. N. (2002). The right brain as the neurobiological substrate of Freud's dynamic unconscious. In D. Scharff (Ed.), *The psychoanalytic century: Freud's legacy for the future* (pp. 61–88). Other Press.

Searls, D. (2017). *The inkblots. Hermann Rorschach, his iconic test, and the power of seeing*. Crown Publishers.

Shapiro, D. (1977). Perceptual understanding of color response. In M. A. Rickers-Osviankina (Ed.), *Rorschach psychology* (pp. 251–301). Robert E. Krieger Publishing CO.

Silberstein, F. (2011). *Etude du modèle théorique du rapport des déterminants de Rorschach par leur comparaison avec une histoire faite avec les réponses* [Study of the theoretical model of the relation of the Rorschach determinants by comparing them with a story made with the answers] [Doctoral dissertation]. Université Lumière Lyon 2.

Silva, D. (2016). Relação entre cor e produção de respostas no Rorschach: Implicações [Relation between color and production of responses in Rorschach: Some implications]. *Revista Iberoamericana de Diagnóstico y Evaluación Psicológica, 1*(41), 174–181. https://www.redalyc.org/jatsRepo/4596/459646901015/html/index.html

Villemor-Amaral, A. E. de (2014). *As pirâmides coloridas de Pfister. Versão para crianças e adolescentes* [Pfister's colored pyramids. Version for children and adolescents]. Casa do Psicólogo/Pearson.

Wundt, W. (1910). *Principles of physiological psychology*. Macmillan.

Yazigi, L. (1995). *A prova de Rorschach, a especialização hemisférica e a epilepsia* [The Rorschach Test, hemispheric specialization and epilepsy] [Postdoctoral thesis]. Departamento de Psiquiatria, Escola Paulista de Medicina, Universidade Federal de São Paulo.

Zeki, S., & Bartels, A. (1999). The clinical and functional measurement of cortical (in) activity in the visual brain, with special reference to the two subdivisions (V4 and V4α) of the human colour centre. *Philosophical Transactions of the Royal Society of London. Series B: Biological Sciences, 354*(1387), 1371–1382. https://doi.org/10.1098/rstb.1999.0485

Zeki, S., & Marini, L. (1998). Three cortical stages of colour processing in the human brain. *Brain, 121*, 1669–1685. https://doi.org/10.1093/brain/121.9.1669

History
Received August 3, 2018
Revision received October 26, 2021
Accepted February 22, 2022
Published online April 28, 2022

Anna Elisa de Villemor-Amaral
Rua Augusto Cioffi 233 Ap 83
Itatiba, São Paulo
Brazil
aevillemor@gmail.com

Summary

This work stemmed from the interest in finding in the field of psychology, and especially in the field of psychological assessment, the evolution of knowledge about the relationship between color and affection, and the relationships between colors and their affective symbolism. The relationship between color and affection has been part of the field of psychological assessment since Herman Rorschach published *Psychodiagnostics* in 1921. However, several studies show that this relationship had already been established since ancestral times and that Herman Rorschach, in developing his method, used this notion that was already rooted in the human mind. From the historical perspective, studies on psychosis based on paintings, artists, and artistic production appear most prominently in the 1940s and bring important contributions to psychology. From then on, there are more systematic investigations on the preference or rejection of certain colors in personality assessment, first in the graphic tests and then in the works of Pfister, with his colored pyramids, and of Lüsher, with his color test. Thus, two lines of investigation are surmised, one that seeks to understand the reaction to colors in general as correlated to affective reactions and another more focused on understanding the specific links between colors and certain emotions. There are studies in the field of neuroscience that aim to demonstrate the basic relationship between color perception and affective reactions in general. At the same time, in other fields of knowledge such as physiology, anthropology, history, and even linguistics, it was more intensely sought to delineate the universal character of the affective meaning of certain colors, bringing important contributions to psychology and to the assessment of personality. Finally, it is noteworthy that there are several convergences and divergences between the research results that are due to the basic difficulty in conducting studies involving color, since the investigated stimuli vary greatly whether they are printed, projected in the form of a luminous ray, or named, in oral or written form, in addition to the great diversity of manifestations of colors with their numerous shades, intensities, and brightness. Finally, a large number of studies, in many different areas, suggest that a combination of factors related to the quality of the light stimulus and their perception involves both biological and cultural aspects that have psychological impact and provide some support for their interpretations and responses to the colored stimulus, but the theme is not exhausted, and there is much yet to be explored.

Resumo

Esse trabalho surgiu do interesse de buscar, no campo da Psicologia e especialmente no da Avaliação Psicológica, a evolução do conhecimento sobre a relação entre cor e afeto, e das relações entre as cores e seus simbolismos afetivos. A relação entre cor e afeto faz parte do campo da Avaliação Psicológica desde que Herman Rorschach publicou seu Psicodiagnóstico em 1921. Porém, diversos estudos demonstram que esta relação já estava estabelecida desde tempos ancestrais e que Herman Rorschach, ao desenvolver seu método, utilizou essa noção já enraizada na mente humana. Do ponto de vista histórico, estudos sobre a pintura, sobre os artistas e sobre a produção artística nos quadros psicóticos aparecem com mais destaque na década de 1940 e trazem contribuições importantes para a Psicologia. A partir de então, encontram-se investigações mais sistemáticas sobre a preferência ou rejeição por determinadas cores na avaliação da personalidade, primeiramente nos testes gráficos e, em seguida, nas obras de Pfister com suas pirâmides coloridas e de Lüsher com seu teste das cores. Assim, depreende-se duas linhas de investigação, uma que busca compreender a reação às cores de um modo geral como correlata às reações afetivas e outra, mais voltada para a compreensão das ligações específicas entre cores e determinadas emoções. Verificam-se, então, estudos no campo das neurociências que visam demonstrar a relação básica entre a percepção das cores e as reações afetivas de um modo geral. Paralelamente, é em outros campos do conhecimento, tais como Fisiologia, Antropologia, História e mesmo Linguística que se buscou mais intensamente deslindar o caráter universal do significado afetivo de determinadas cores, trazendo igualmente contribuições importantes para a Psicologia e para a avaliação da personalidade. Destaca-se finalmente que há diversas convergências e divergências entre os resultados das pesquisas e que isso se deve à dificuldade básica na condução de estudos envolvendo cor, uma vez que os estímulos investigados variam muito se são impressos, se são projetados na forma de raio luminoso ou se são nomeados, na forma oral ou escrita, além da grande diversidade de manifestações das cores com suas inúmeras tonalidades, intensidades e brilho. Finalmente, a grande quantidade de estudos, nas mais diferentes áreas, sugere que uma combinação de fatores relacionados às qualidades do estímulo luminoso e sua percepção, envolve tanto aspectos biológicos quanto culturais, que repercutem psicologicamente e dão certa sustentação para as interpretações às respostas ao estímulo colorido, mas o tema não se esgota, havendo muito ainda a ser explorado.

Résumé

Ce travail est né de l'intérêt de rechercher, dans le domaine de la psychologie et en particulier dans le domaine de l'évaluation psychologique, l'évolution des connaissances sur la relation entre la couleur et l'affection, et des relations entre les couleurs et leurs symbolismes affectifs. La relation entre la couleur et l'affection fait partie du champ de l'évaluation psychologique depuis qu'Herman Rorschach a publié son Psychodiagnostic en 1921. Cependant, plusieurs études démontrent que cette relation est établie depuis l'Antiquité et qu'Herman Rorschach, lors du développement de sa méthode, a utilisé cette notion déjà enracinée dans l'esprit humain. D'un point de vue historique, les études sur la peinture, sur les artistes et sur la production artistique de psychotiques apparaissent plus en évidence dans les années 1940 et apportent des contributions importantes à la psychologie. Dès lors, des investigations plus systématiques sur la préférence ou le rejet de certaines couleurs se retrouvent dans l'évaluation de la personnalité, d'abord dans les tests graphiques puis dans les œuvres de Pfister avec ses pyramides colorées et Lüsher avec son test de couleur. Ainsi, deux pistes d'investigation émergent, l'une qui cherche à comprendre la réaction aux couleurs de manière générale comme corrélée aux réactions affectives et l'autre, plus focalisée sur la compréhension des liens spécifiques entre les couleurs et certaines émotions. Ensuite, il y a des études dans le domaine des neurosciences qui visent à démontrer la relation de base entre la perception des couleurs et les réactions affectives en général. Dans le même temps, c'est dans d'autres domaines de la connaissance, tels que la physiologie, l'anthropologie, l'histoire et même la linguistique, que nous avons cherché plus intensément à démêler le caractère universel de la signification affective de certaines couleurs, apportant également des contributions importantes à la psychologie et à l'évaluation de la personnalité. Enfin, il est à noter qu'il existe plusieurs convergences et divergences entre les résultats de la recherche et que cela est dû à la difficulté fondamentale à mener des études impliquant la couleur, puisque les stimuli étudiés varient beaucoup s'ils sont imprimés, s'ils sont projetés sous la forme d'un rayon lumineux ou qu'ils soient nommés, sous forme orale ou écrite, en plus de la grande diversité des manifestations de couleur avec leurs nombreuses nuances, intensités et brillances. Enfin, le grand nombre d'études, dans les domaines les plus différents, suggère qu'une combinaison de facteurs liés aux qualités du stimulus lumineux et à sa perception, implique à la fois des aspects biologiques et culturels, qui ont un impact psychologique et apportent un certain soutien aux interprétations des réponses au stimulus colorées, mais le thème ne s'arrête pas, il reste encore beaucoup à explorer.

Resumen

Este trabajo surge del interés de buscar, en el campo de la Psicología y especialmente en el campo de la Evaluación Psicológica, la evolución del conocimiento sobre la relación entre color y afecto, y de las relaciones entre los colores y sus simbolismos afectivos. La relación entre color y afecto ha sido parte del campo de la Evaluación Psicológica desde que Herman Rorschach publicó su Psicodiagnóstico en 1921. Sin embargo, varios estudios demuestran que esta relación se ha establecido desde la antigüedad y que Herman Rorschach, al desarrollar su método, utilizó esta noción ya arraigada en la mente humana. Desde un punto de vista histórico, los estudios sobre pintura, sobre artistas y sobre producción artística en cuadros psicóticos aparecen de forma más destacada en la década de 1940 y aportan importantes contribuciones a la Psicología. A partir de entonces, las investigaciones más sistemáticas sobre la preferencia o rechazo de determinados colores se encuentran en evaluación de la personalidad, primero en las pruebas gráficas y luego en las obras de Pfister con sus pirámides coloreadas y de Lüsher con su prueba de colores. Así, surgen dos líneas de investigación, una que busca comprender la reacción a los colores de manera general como correlacionada con las reacciones afectivas y la otra, más enfocada a comprender los vínculos específicos entre los colores y determinadas emociones. Luego, hay estudios en el campo de las neurociencias que tienen como objetivo demostrar la relación básica entre la percepción del color y las reacciones afectivas en general. Al mismo tiempo, es en otros campos del conocimiento, como la Fisiología, la Antropología, la Historia e incluso la Lingüística, donde se buscó con más intensidad desentrañar el carácter universal del significado afectivo de ciertos colores, aportando también importantes aportes a la Psicología y a la evaluación de la personalidad. Finalmente, es de destacar que existen varias convergencias y divergencias entre los resultados de las investigaciones y que esto se debe a la dificultad básica de realizar estudios que involucren el color, ya que los estímulos investigados varían mucho si se imprimen, si se proyectan como rayo de luz o si se nombran, de forma oral o escrita, además de la gran diversidad de manifestaciones cromáticas con sus numerosos matices, intensidades y brillos. Finalmente, la gran cantidad de estudios, en las áreas más diferentes, sugiere que una combinación de factores relacionados con las cualidades del estímulo lumínico y su percepción involucra aspectos tanto biológicos como culturales, que tienen un impacto psicológico y brindan algún apoyo a las interpretaciones de las respuestas al estímulo coloridas, pero el tema no termina, aún queda mucho por explorar.

要約

本論文は、心理学の分野、特に心理アセスメントの分野で、色彩と感情との関係、色彩とその感情の象徴的な側面に関する知見の展開に興味を持ったことに端を発している。色彩と感情との関係は、1921年にヘルマン・ロールシャッハが「精神診断学」を出版して以来、心理アセスメントの一部となっている。しかし、この関係はすでに先祖代々から確立されたものであり、ヘルマン・ロールシャッハがその手法を開発する時に、すでに人間の心に根ざしていた概念を用いていたことが、いくつかの研究で示されている。歴史的に見ると、絵画、や画家、芸術作品に基づく精神病の研究は、1940年代に最も顕著に現れ、心理学に重要な貢献をもたらした。それ以後、グラフィックテスト、フィスターのカラーピラミッド、リュッシャーのカラーテストなど、パーソナリティアセスメントにおける特定の色の選択や拒否に関する研究がより体系的に行われるようになっていった。このように、色に対する反応全般を感情的な反応として理解しようとするものと、色と特定の感情との関係理解することに焦点づけられたものの、2つの研究の流れが想定される。神経科学の分野では、色彩知覚と感情反応全般の基本的な関係を明らかにすることを目的とした研究がある。一方、生理学、人類学、歴史学さらには言語学など他の知識分野では、ある色が持つ感情的な意味の普遍性を明らかにすることがより強く求められ、心理学やパーソナリティの評価に重要な貢献をもたらした。最後に、色彩研究は基本的には難しいが、それは色彩が印刷されたものだったり、光線として投影されたものだったり、口頭や文字で名付けられていたり、またその濃淡や強弱、明るさなど多様な表出をするため、研究結果の間にいくつかの収束と拡散があることに注目すべきである。そして、光刺激の質とその知覚に関する要因の組み合わせには、心理的な影響を及ぼす生物学的および文化的な側面が含まれ、色刺激に対する解釈や反応における多くの研究において示唆されているが、このテーマはまだ尽きておらず、まだ解明されていないことも多い。

Book Review

Hermann Rorschach's Psychodiagnostics (2021)

Filippo Aschieri

Rorschach, H. (2021)
Hermann Rorschach's Psychodiagnostics:
Newly Translated and Annotated 100ᵗʰ Anniversary Edition
(P. J. Keddy, R. Signer, P. Erdberg, &
A. Schneider-Stocking, Trans. & Eds.)
(Original published in 1921)
Hogrefe Publishing, 294 pages
ISBN (Print) 978-0-88937-558-1, US $69.00, € 59.95
ISBN (PDF) 978-1-61676-558-3, US $59.99, € 52.99
https://doi.org/10.1027/00558-000

One century after its first edition, the Rorschach Test is still developing, both in its scoring methods and in its fields of application (Mihura et al., 2022). What John Exner wrote in 1969, a few years before the first edition of the Comprehensive System (1974) about the presence of many Rorschach systems that have in common only the 10 cards, still holds true today. Since 1921, Rorschach systems have varied increasingly in terms of the response coding and of the rationale underlying the test itself. Comparative examinations of Rorschach methods show their differences in theoretical and empirical backgrounds (Prudent et al., 2022), particularly between psychodynamic and empirical approaches (Aschieri & Pascarella, 2021; Guinzbourg de Braude et al., 2021; Meskanen & Pucci, 2021).

Thus, in 2022, a reading of *Hermann Rorschach's Psychodiagnostics*, translated and edited by Philip J. Keddy, Rita Signer, Philip Erdberg, and Arianna Schneider-Stocking and published by Hogrefe in 2021, could be particularly enlightening for returning to the test origins and rationale with fresh eyes. This book contains the new translation of the original text by Hermann Rorschach, but it is much more than that.

In fact, the authors include additional relevant material that goes well beyond the translation of the book. Readers have access to the biography of Hermann

Rorschach, an analysis of the writings that preceded the 1921 book, a translation of a lecture by Hermann Rorschach on the relationship between the test and psychoanalysis that was published right after the publication of the book, a glossary collecting the terms used in the translation, a list of publications from Hermann Rorschach, and a section on the annotations to the translation. The amount of material included in this volume speaks of the monumental effort made by the authors to provide readers with the most complete, accurate, and up-to-date publication possible.

The biography and the subsequent sections, written by Rita Signer, probably one of the best contemporary experts on Hermann Rorschach (see, e.g., Müller & Signer, 2004; Signer & Müller, 2005, 2008) present a fresh, detailed, and vivid description of Hermann Rorschach's life, personality, and thinking. Signer reports the influence of Jung in his studies, his psychoanalytic writings, and the trajectory of his career from his first position in a psychiatric hospital close to Bern to the role of associate director at the psychiatric hospital in Herisau. However, most notably, readers will feel the spirit with which Rorschach devoted himself to clinical work, developing a test that would eventually become a great tool for exploring "the most interesting thing in nature [which] is the human soul" (p. 16), and be the basis for therapeutic assessment, since the "highest thing a person can do is to heal sick souls" (Müller & Signer, p. 8, in Rorschach, 1921/2021, p. 16).

The section on "The Creation of Psychodiagnostics" describes the background of the creation of the test and provides wonderful examples of the ambiguous images that accompanied the development of the inkblots. It offers readers a description of the work that Hermann Rorschach did "behind the scenes" prior to the publication of *Psychodiagnostics* in 1921: from the initial experiment conducted in 1911 with students, to the refinements of the "perceptual-diagnostic experiment" he wrote about in 1918, 1919, and 1920. Signer provides a summary of the 1918 text on *Investigations on Perception and Apperception in Healthy and Ill Persons: Draft*, giving the readers an introduction to how inkblots were made, and how the author initially tested the "concurrent validity" of movement color determinants, using ambiguous drawings· along with the inkblots. The section also reports on the rationale of the perception and apperception processes measured by Hermann Rorschach's experiment.

In the summary of the first 1919 text, *On Perception and Apperception in Healthy and Ill Persons* (Rorschach, 1919a), Signer highlights the growing interest of Hermann Rorschach in the curvilinear relationship between Rorschach movement and introversion tendencies. He found that the more intelligent and resourceful respondents were, the more movements they had in their responses to the test. However, the presence of movements was also correlated with extremely introverted respondents. Extreme cases of introversion were representative of patients suffering from autism. Signer highlighted, based on documenting Rorschach's reading of the *Essai sur l'introversion mystique* written by the psychiatrist Ferdinand Morel (1918), the influences on Hermann Rorschach's view of introversion by Janet, Bleuer, and Jung concepts of reality function, autism, and introversion, which were extensively cited in Morel's book.

In the summary of the second text from 1919, *A Perceptual-Diagnostic Experiment* (Rorschach, 1919b), Signer stresses a development in the definition of the "experience type." Rorschach clarified the relation of extratensive and intratensive respondents with color and movement responses (Rorschach, 1921/2021):

> On the one hand, the "color influences" stand in direct proportion to the extraversive factors; yet on the other hand, they stand in direct proportion to the lability of affects. Kinesthesias are, on the one hand, in direct proportion to the introversive factors; yet, on the other hand, they are in direct proportion to the stability of affects. (p. 26)

Signer finally addresses the main points and developments that appeared in the last text prior to the publication of the manual, titled *A Perceptual-Diagnostic Experiment* (1920). In this text, Hermann Rorschach further clarified that, "there is no introverted and extraverted type, but only a predominantly introverted one capable of introversions, as well as a predominantly extraverted one capable of extraversion" (Rorschach, 1920, p. 14, in Rorschach, 1921/2021, p. 25). Not only are extraversion and introversion dynamic categories of individual functioning, but in this text Hermann Rorschach stressed the possibility of changing the predominant approach during one's lifetime, and that these categories could also be used to describe cultural periods and changes at a societal level.

The central part of the newly published volume is devoted to the new translation of the Hermann Rorschach masterpiece *Psychodiagnostics* (1921), which is presented in a fresh, relatable, and clear language. Some translation choices, among many, are worth mentioning. For example, the previously used "modes of apperception" are now referred to as "modes of visual grasping," and some headings of paragraphs were re-edited to provide a more informative description of the contents of the text going beyond the "single word" title originally used by the author. A noteworthy surprise is the use of "plates" instead of "cards" to refer to the support of the inkblots.

Other changes to the previous translation of the book are connected to "hints" added by the translators with the aim of facilitating the readers' use of the book. For example, the responses of the 28 Rorschach protocols included in the book have been numbered, facilitating (a) the understanding of how Hermann

Rorschach defined the boundaries of Rorschach responses and (b) the understanding of his coding.

After the main text, the editors have also translated the paper titled "The Evaluation of the Form Interpretation Experiment for Psychoanalysis" – already presented in the 1942 English edition of *Psychodiagnostics*. In this section it is particularly interesting to observe how Hermann Rorschach systematically proceeded in the interpretation of a real protocol, moving from smaller inferences based on individual variables (or groups of variables), to corroborating inferences comparing indications from different typologies of variables, to framing such inferences within relevant theoretical backgrounds.

A reader studying this content should already feel enriched and fulfilled at this point in the book. Remarkably, however, the editors have added even more content that is extremely useful for readers: a glossary of key terms used by Hermann Rorschach in *Psychodiagnostics*, the complete list of publications by (and on) Hermann Rorschach, and finally the uniquely valuable annotations to the translation of the book contents. These annotations would be worthy of a publication in and of themselves because they provide theoretical background to "concepts" that were widely known at the beginning of the last century and that might be harder to grasp today. For example, terms such as those that appear in the following passage would remain obscure to most readers without the care that the editors took to guide the readers in the historical background of the volume (Rorschach, 1921/2021):

> Rorschach cites Eugen Bleuler's idea of perception from the latter's *Lehrbuch der Psychiatrie* (*Textbook of Psychiatry*; Bleuler, 1916, p. 9). For Bleuler, perception consisted of three components: sensation, memory, and association. Rorschach deduced that the "interpretations" of his klecksographies were "doubtlessly" perceptions, yet with one difference: all perceptions "identifying integrations between sensation-complexes are memories of sensation-complexes." These "integrations" occur "unconsciously" during everyday perceptions. However, in the experiment, the incongruence between sensation-complexes and memories of sensation-complexes are [sic] so great that this effort of integration is perceived intrapsychically as an effort by the respondents. (p. 21)

Also, these annotations allow us to make sense of some examples used by Hermann Rorschach that today would probably be hard to understand. For example, I found fascinating the use of King Wilhelm II and Luis XIV as prototypical examples of extratensive personalities, without reference to narcissism, which is now a feature reliably measured by the test (Mihura et al., 2013).

In conclusion, I would strongly recommend this book to all Rorschach users. It provides a description of Hermann Rorschach and of the cultural and scientific background in which the test was created, and is written in a language adapted to contemporary psychological thinking. An active reading of the book will be a test for our own view of psychopathology and our own ability to adapt Rorschach concepts to contemporary psychology.

References

Aschieri, F., & Pascarella, G. (2021). A systematic narrative review of evaluating change in psychotherapy with the Rorschach test. *Rorschachiana, 42*(2), 232–257. https://doi.org/10.1027/1192-5604/a000142

Bleuler, E. (1916). *Lehrbuch der Psychiatrie* [Textbook of psychiatry]. Springer.

Exner, J. E. (1969). *The Rorschach systems*. Grune & Stratton.

Exner, J. E. (1974). *The Rorschach: A comprehensive system*. Wiley.

Guinzbourg de Braude, S. M., Vibert, S., Righetti, T., & Antonelli, A. (2021). Eating disorders and the Rorschach: A research review from the French School and the Comprehensive System. *Rorschachiana, 42*(2), 202–224. https://doi.org/10.1027/1192-5604/a000136

Meskanen, K., & Pucci, M. (2021). A commentary on "Eating disorders and the Rorschach" (Guinzbourg de Braude et al., 2021). *Rorschachiana, 42*(2), 225–231. https://doi.org/10.1027/1192-5604/a000148

Mihura, J. L., Jowers, C. E., Dumitrascu, N., Villanueva van den Hurk, A. W., & Keddy, P. J. (2022). The specific uses of the Rorschach in clinical practice: Preliminary results from an international survey. *Rorschachiana, 43*(1), 25–41. https://doi.org/10.1027/1192-5604/a000155.

Mihura, J. L., Meyer, G. J., Dumitrascu, N., & Bombel, G. (2013). The validity of individual Rorschach variables: Systematic reviews and meta-analyses of the comprehensive system. *Psychological Bulletin, 139*(3), 548–605. https://doi.org/10.1037/a0029406

Morel, F. (1918). *Essai sur l'introversion mystique: étude psychologique de Pseudo-Denys l'Areopagite et de quelques autres cas de mysticisme* [Essay on mystical introversion: A psychological study of Pseudo-Denys the Areopagite and some other cases of mysticism]. Kundig.

Müller, C. & Signer, R. (Eds.). (2004). *Hermann Rorschach (1884–1922): Briefwechsel: Ausgewählt und herausgegeben von Christian Müller und Rita Signer* [Correspondence: Selected and edited by Christian Müller and Rita Signer]. Verlag Hans Huber.

Prudent, C., Kleiger, J., Husain, O., & De Tychey, C. (2022). On psychosis: An international comparative single case study of the Nancy French, Lausanne, and American Rorschach approaches. *Rorschachiana, 43*(1), 42–69. https://doi.org/10.1027/1192-5604/a000151

Rorschach, H. (1918). *Untersuchungen über die Wahrnehmung und Auffassung bei Gesunden und Kranken, Entwurf* [Investigations on perception and apperception in healthy and ill persons, draft] (Rorsch HR 3:3:6:1). Hermann Rorschach Archive, Institute for the History of Medicine, Bern, Switzerland.

Rorschach, H. (1919a). *Zur Wahrnehmung und Auffassung bei Gesunden und Kranken* [On perception and apperception in healthy and ill persons] [Typewritten lecture manuscript] (Rorsch HR 3:2:1:1). Hermann Rorschach Archive, Institute for the History of Medicine, Bern, Switzerland.

Rorschach, H. (1919b). *Ein wahrnehmungsdiagnostisches Experiment* [A perceptual-diagnostic experiment] [Typewritten lecture manuscript] (Rorsch HR 3:2:1:2). Hermann Rorschach Archive, Institute for the History of Medicine, Bern, Switzerland.

Rorschach, H. (1920). *Ein wahrnehmungs-diagnostischer Versuch* [A perceptual-diagnostic experiment] [Typewritten lecture manuscript] (Rorsch HR 3:2:1:3). Hermann Rorschach Archive, Institute for the History of Medicine, Bern, Switzerland.

Rorschach, H. (1921). *Psychodiagnostik: Methodik und Ergebnisse eines wahrnehmungs-diagnostischen Experiments (Deutenlassen von Zufallsformen)* [Psychodiagnostics: methodology and results of a perceptual-diagnostic experiment (eliciting interpretations of accidental forms)]. Bircher.

Rorschach, H. (2021). *Hermann Rorschach's psychodiagnostics: Newly translated and annotated 100th anniversary edition* (P. J. Keddy, R. Signer, P. Erdberg, & A. Schneider-Stocking, Trans. & Eds.). Hogrefe Publishing. (Original work published 1921)

Signer, R., & Müller, C. (2005). Was liest ein Psychiater zu Beginn des 20. Jahrhunderts? Die Fachlektüre Hermann Rorschachs im Kontext seiner psychiatrischen und wissenschaftlichen Tätigkeit [What does a psychiatrist read at the beginning of the 20th century? Hermann Rorschach's scientific reading in the context of his professional practice and scientific activity]. *Schweizer Archiv für Neurologie und Psychiatrie, 156*(6), 279–284. https://doi.org/10.4414/sanp.2005.01623

Signer, R., & Müller, C. (2008). „Ich will nie mehr … nur Bücher lesen, sondern Menschen". Die Entstehungsgeschichte des Rorschach-Tests ["I never want to read … just books again, but people." The genesis of the Rorschach Test]. In I. Blum & P. Witschi (Eds.), *Olga und Hermann Rorschach. Ein ungewöhnliches Psychiater-Ehepaar* (pp. 13–23). Appenzeller.

Published online April 28, 2022

ORCID
Filippo Aschieri
https://orcid.org/0000-0002-1164-5926

Filippo Aschieri
European Center for Therapeutic Assessment
Università Cattolica del Sacro Cuore
L.go Gemelli 1
20123 Milan
Italy
filippo.aschieri@unicatt.it

Editorial

Searching for a Common Language to Talk About the Rorschach Within and Outside the International Society of the Rorschach and Projective Methods

Filippo Aschieri

European Center for Therapeutic Assessment, Università Cattolica del Sacro Cuore, Milan, Italy

The Christian saying, "A couple that prays together stays together," suggests that when couples pray together, they open a dialogue with a third entity (God) that allows the partners to increase their mutual understanding and intimacy. King and colleagues (2022) recently provided empirical support for this saying. In a 10-year longitudinal study with 371 families, they found that couples with higher levels of religiosity engaged in more joint activities over time. Shared beliefs, common wishes, and similar values improved couples' functioning, and increased the quality of their relationship. In the International Society of the Rorschach and Projective Methods (ISR) we all revere the Rorschach, and our common beliefs are around the value of "facilitate[ing] scientific exchanges among specialists, practitioners and researchers in the field" (ISR bylaws, Article 1). But what kind of "common praying" should the ISR do to "stay together"? What would help the subgroups within our larger group understand each other? What would help the ISR to increase cohesion internally and improve its impact externally?

Historically, cohesion has been considered the most important variable in groups (Lott & Lott, 1965), and – even though its definition has been controversial – a comprehensive meta-analysis stressed that both social cohesion (e.g., hanging out at gala dinners in congresses) and task cohesion (e.g., working together to improve the quality of the services the ISR provides for its members) are fundamental for a group to effectively tackle its challenges (Chiocchio & Essiembre, 2009).

Since 2021, the current editorial board decided to promote cohesion in the ISR by offering its members occasions for "thinking together" about the Rorschach. My hope is that this issue of *Rorschachiana* will also represent an occasion to promote community dialogue on the Rorschach. Community dialogue has been defined as "an interactive, community-based planning process that brings together participants from different sections of a community and encourages them to think about, discuss and explore underlying issues of concern" (Bernstein & Isaac, 2021,

Rorschachiana (2022), 43(2), 95–102
https://doi.org/10.1027/1192-5604/a000159

p. 2). Community dialogue fosters community engagement in socially relevant issues, improves common understanding of problems, and has a positive impact on people's sense of connection, belonging, and trust in the group (DeTurk, 2006; Frantell et al., 2019).

Building community dialogue requires finding a common language to use in discourse. The 2021 special issue, dedicated to the centenary of the publication of *Psychodiagnosis* (Rorschach, 1921), aimed at promoting dialogue between members of the ISR and between the Rorschach community and the wider professional audience by providing updated reviews of research in specific fields of study and application of the Rorschach test (Carstairs, 2021), each commented on by experts in the field.

The goal proved to be ambitious, certainly successful but not without difficulties. On the one hand, it seems that "within" the Rorschach community, languages can be very different and may get in the way of promoting communication and mutual understanding. This was highlighted, for example, by the commentary of Meskanen and Pucci (2021) to Guinzbourg de Braude and colleagues' article (2021) on the use of Rorschach with eating disorders. Meskanen and Pucci (2021) stressed that results using the CS and the French Rorschach approach are difficult integrate and synthesize. Similarly, different research methods used in Rorschach research can greatly complicate the task of summarizing and understanding research results. The commentary made by Andre van Graan (2021) on the paper on neurobiology (Jimura et al., 2021) highlighted how the variety of methods used to inspect the neurobiological correlates of the test makes it harder today, if not impossible, to accumulate research and replicate findings across studies. Finally, perspectives of Rorschach users of the qualities of the test may sound overly positive to the larger professional community. For example, the commentary of Hopwood and colleagues (2021), based on the demanding criteria of psychotherapy research, "toned down" the perhaps overly positive conclusions of Aschieri and Pascarella (2021) with regard to the quality of the Rorschach as a measure of psychotherapy outcome. The unfortunate conclusion is: We, as Rorschach users, are not very capable of talking with each other, and when we open up a dialogue with professionals from other fields, we may find that it is not easy to attune to external standards of research quality.

The current issue, originally envisioned by Sadegh Nashat and myself, is an effort to advance a common language to talk about the Rorschach both with Rorschach users and with non-Rorschach users in two ways. The first, is by offering the first keynote speech of the Geneva Congress by Robert Bornstein in the form of an Invited Keynote Address (Bornstein, 2022). The author provides a detailed and encompassing response to the crucial question, "What is the Rorschach test?," and describes the impact that Rorschach-based science can have on psychodiagnosis and on the field of psychology at large. The second is by focusing the issue, through three articles, on "New insights from other psychological disciplines for Rorschach users."

The first article, written by Meyer and Friston (2022) represents a ground-breaking application of the Bayesian model of the mind to the Rorschach test. The other two articles from Christman (2022) and Capelli and colleagues (2022) deal, respectively, with the impact of the lateralization process on Rorschach responses, and with the psychological functions and processes connected to skin contact in children and adults.

Meyer and Friston's (2022) paper brings a breath of fresh air to the task of answering the question: "Why is the Rorschach test useful?" As an answer, their paper includes a short and clear summary of more than a decade of neurobiology studies that advocate for the brain's active role in shaping perception to minimize the difference between the expected and actual sensory input. The most basic function of the brain, in this perspective, is to recursively (1) predict the environment and the sensations it should provide, (2) record the sensations received from the environment, (3) act to sample further if the "categorization" is accurate, and (4) update the prediction of the environment if the action signals back that the environment did not fit with the prior expectations. More "sophisticated" functions include the anticipation of future mismatch between actual and expected input depending on different courses of action. The Rorschach test, in this framework, is probably the best possible way to "picture" what each person thinks (anticipates) of their environment and what each person does (in Rorschach terms – what each person projects or attributes to the stimulus or behaves or performs – depending on the system used) to adapt to the "environment" represented by the card. According to the authors, the Rorschach test "provides an unprecedented tool to explore the landscape of a subject's prior beliefs about the causes of their sensations. In one sense, Rorschach's task is the ultimate tool for disclosing prior beliefs" (Meyer & Friston, 2022, p. 138), as "Rorschach recognized the task, while one of perception, also helped show the iterative cycle of prediction, error correction, active search, revised prediction, further error correction, further action, and so on" (p. 139). The authors detail how various features of the test coding and response processes, such as movement, ideation, and form distortion, can be illuminated by this perspective, and – most notably – how the recent translation of Hermann Rorschach's book (Rorschach, 1921/2021) showed clear overlaps in the understanding of these phenomena between Rorschach himself and the "Bayesian" view of the mind.

This article should interest psychoanalytic Rorschach users as it gives a new and empirically supported meaning to the concept of "projection" onto the cards. Similarly, could the Bayesian concepts of active anticipation and of action be effective ways to "translate" concepts of transference to the assessor and of projective identification? Clinicians interested in therapeutic and collaborative assessment are also potentially interested in this manuscript, due to the implications this view of the mind has on what "therapy" should be. For example, if the Rorschach helps us understand what clients expect regarding problematic emotional states, then the Rorschach extended inquiry (Fantini et al., 2022) can be used both to highlight those expectations and to aid clients' Bayesian brain to adjust expectations based on "here and now" sensorial feedback in the assessor–client relationship. This view further supports the well-known importance of the assessor's active role in disconfirming the client's pathogenetic expectations based on their previous negative relational experiences – and showed by the testing – during a therapeutic or collaborative assessment.

Christman's paper (2022) is a powerful reminder of how much we still do not know about the Rorschach. While a few recent studies on adults ruled out the existence of significant Rorschach differences connected to age, gender, and ethnicity (Meyer et al., 2015), it is surprising to discover the potential for biased interpretations of the test results depending on other factors such as the hemispheric dominance. My hope is that this paper will revive an exciting field of study for Rorschach users: Does hemispheric dominance impact differently Rorschach results? If significant differences were found, would they imply the need for specific norms depending on the outcome of the lateralization process and the stability versus nonstability of hemispheric dominance? This paper is also of the utmost importance for all forensic psychologists, who may want to include in their reports that their test interpretations are mindful of the clients' hemisphere dominance.

Capelli and colleagues (2022) offer a summary of the psychological functions that are organized around the skin contact in children and adults. Through skin contact, for example, caregivers actively contribute to their infants' sense of body ownership and self–other differentiation; improve children's emotional regulation; promote cognitive abilities such as sustained attention, object exploration, and delay of gratification; and improve brain maturation and the overall healthy development of the child. Since Anzieu's conceptualization of "skin ego" (1989), Rorschach users proposed the test as a useful tool to infer the quality of the internalized representations of contact. Unfortunately, the research background to these inferences is not as solid as the empirical correlates of the skin contact with early and mature caregivers appearing in Capelli and colleagues' paper (2022). Instead, Fisher and Cleveland (1958) developed the Barrier and Penetration (BP) scoring system in the Rorschach as a means to reliably and objectively measure respondents' body image and the quality of body boundaries. The authors (Fisher & Cleveland, 1968) assumed that:

Definiteness of boundaries is linked with the ability to be an independent person who has definite standards, definite goals, and forceful, striving ways of approaching tasks. We visualized the person with definite boundaries as one who sought special success in life and as one who could not easily be diverted by stress or obstacles from goal attainment. We pictured boundary definiteness as carrying with it a facility for expressing tension by attacking and shaping the environment to make it conform to the individual's internalized standards. (p. 117)

Barrier responses include images in which "emphasis [is] on the definite structure, substance, and surface qualities of boundaries" (O'Neill, 2005, p. 162). Penetration responses include images featured by "weakness, lack of substance, and penetrability" (ibid).

O'Neill (2005) summarized the main findings of more than 100 studies on BP focusing on coding reliability (excellent for both dimensions), temporal stability (very high), gender differences, age differences, and validity. In general, women tend to have more Barrier (8 responses vs. 7) and less Penetration (2 responses vs. 3) responses than men. Less consistent results emerge when considering the effect of age on Barrier and Penetration responses, which in some cases seems to be positively correlated (Fisher, 1986), while other studies found more Barrier and Penetration responses in younger respondents than in protocols from adults and older adults (Hayslip et al., 1997).

In terms of validity, Fisher and Cleveland (1968) concluded their summary of the first 15 years of research on this scale that BP responses have distinct correlation patterns: Barrier scores are generally predictable and consistent, while Penetration scores are valid only when measured with "extreme" groups of respondents. This finding limited the research on Penetration scores, and most of the subsequent studies focused on Barrier responses. O'Neill's review (2005) of BP research concluded that:

High-Barrier individuals would be more self-steering. Specifically, they found that individuals with more definite boundaries had higher achievement motivation, set more ambitious goals for themselves, had a greater desire for task completion, were less suggestible, made fewer errors on stressful tasks, and more realistically adjusted to task-performance failure. Interpersonally, they were more likely to communicate with others, and were more interested in careers involving people rather than things. (p. 173)

The study by Capelli and colleagues (2022) provides an updated conceptual background to sustain the importance of touch as the basis of a healthy psychological development. BP scores – to date – appear to be an interesting coding system for linking empirical connections between these concepts and the Rorschach. In particular, the first goal would be to complete a systematic literature review on BP. Second, BP coding categories should be refined to avoid overlaps with other established codes, such as MOR contents (O'Neill, 2005). Finally, and perhaps most importantly, BP responses should also include other features beside the actual content, such as form quality and other special scores that may impact their interpretation. As suggested by various manuals of Rorschach interpretation (Exner, 2003; Meyer et al., 2011) clinicians should not limit the interpretation of Texture response to their raw number, but also evaluate their quality (i.e., a "hard rock" would necessarily be interpreted differently from "soft fur").

Back to this volume, I believe that human existence "is not in minds but in meetings" (Cissna & Anderson, 2002, p. 17), and so I hope readers of this issue will find the desire to increase occasions for sharing and discussing topics such as, "What the Rorschach test is," and about how to use it at its best. Hopefully, this approach will provide our Society with a meeting space both to keep informed about the latest topics of our interest, and also to promote creativity and cohesion within the community.

References

Andre van Graan, L. (2021). A commentary on "Can neuroscience provide a new foundation for the Rorschach variables?" (Jimura et al., 2021). *Rorschachiana, 42*(2), 166–174. https://doi.org/10.1027/1192-5604/a000149

Anzieu, D. (1989). *The skin ego: A psychoanalytic approach to the self* (C Turner, Trans.). Yale University Press.

Aschieri, F., & Pascarella, G. (2021). A systematic narrative review of evaluating change in psychotherapy with the Rorschach test. *Rorschachiana, 42*(2), 232–257. https://doi.org/10.1027/1192-5604/a000142

Bernstein, A. G., & Isaac, C. A. (2021). Gentrification: The role of dialogue in community engagement and social cohesion. *Journal of Urban Affairs.* Advance online publication. https://doi.org/10.1080/07352166.2021.1877550

Bornstein, R. (2022). Toward an integrative perspective on the person: Using Rorschach data to enhance the diagnostic systems. *Rorschachiana, 43*(2), 103–127.

Capelli, E., Grumi, S., Fullone, E., Rinaldi, E., & Provenzi, L. (2022). An update on social touch: How does humans' social nature emerge at the periphery of the body? *Rorschachiana, 43*(2), 168–185. https://doi.org/10.1027/1192-5604/a000153

Carstairs, K. (2021). Celebrating 100 Years. *Rorschachiana, 42*(2), 113–117. https://doi.org/10.1027/1192-5604/a000150

Chiocchio, F., & Essiembre, H. (2009). Cohesion and performance: A meta-analytic review of disparities between project teams, production teams, and service teams. *Small Group Research, 40*(4), 382–420. https://doi.org/10.1177/1046496409335103

Christman, S. (2022). The right hemisphere and ambiguity: A possible role of handedness in Rorschach responsivity. *Rorschachiana, 43*(2), 151–167. https://doi.org/10.1027/1192-5604/a000152

Cissna, K. N., & Anderson, R. (2002). *Moments of meeting: Buber, Rogers, and the potential for public dialogue.* SUNY Press.

DeTurk, S. (2006). The power of dialogue: Consequences of intergroup dialogue and their implications for agency and alliance building. *Communication Quarterly, 54*(1), 33–51. https://doi.org/10.1080/01463370500270355

Exner, J. E. Jr. (2003). *The Rorschach: A Comprehensive System: Vol. 1. Basic foundations and principles of interpretation* (4th ed.). Wiley.

Fantini, F., Aschieri, F., David, R. M., Martin, H., & Finn, S. E. (2022). *Therapeutic assessment with adults: Using psychological testing to help clients change.* Routledge.

Fisher, S. (1986). *Development and structure of the body image* (Vols. 1, 2). Lawrence Erlbaum Associates.

Fisher, S., & Cleveland, S. E. (1958). *Body image and personality.* Van Nostrand.

Fisher, S., & Cleveland, S. E. (1968). *Body image and personality* (2nd ed.). Dover.

Frantell, K. A., Miles, J. R., & Ruwe, A. M. (2019). Intergroup dialogue: A review of recent empirical research and its implications for research and practice. *Small Group Research, 50*(5), 654–695. https://doi.org/10.1177/1046496419835923

Guinzbourg de Braude, S. M., Vibert, S., Righetti, T., & Antonelli, A. (2021). Eating disorders and the Rorschach: A research review from the French school and the comprehensive system. *Rorschachiana, 42*(2), 202–224. https://doi.org/10.1027/1192-5604/a000136

Hayslip, B. Jr., Cooper, C. C., Dougherty, L. M., & Cook, D. B. (1997). Body image in adulthood: A projective approach. *Journal of Personality Assessment, 68*(3), 628–649.

Hopwood, C. J., Yalch, M. M., & Luo, X. (2021). A commentary on "A systematic narrative review of evaluating change in psychotherapy" (Aschieri & Pascarella, 2021): More rigor is needed in research on the Rorschach and treatment change. *Rorschachiana, 42*(2), 258–264. https://doi.org/10.1027/1192-5604/a000146

Jimura, K., Asari, T., & Nakamura, N. (2021). Can neuroscience provide a new foundation for the Rorschach variables? *Rorschachiana, 42*(2), 143–165. https://doi.org/10.1027/1192-5604/a000147

King, V., Wickrama, K. A. S., & Beach, S. R. H. (2022). Religiosity and joint activities of husbands and wives in enduring marriages. *Psychology of Religion and Spirituality, 14*(1), 97–107. https://doi.org/10.1037/rel0000370

Lott, A. J., & Lott, B. E. (1965). Group cohesiveness as interpersonal attraction: A review of relationships with antecedent and consequent variables. *Psychological Bulletin, 64*(4), 259–309. https://doi.org/10.1037/h0022386

Meskanen, K., & Pucci, M. (2021). A commentary on "Eating disorders and the Rorschach" (Guinzbourg de Braude et al., 2021). *Rorschachiana, 42*(2), 225–231. https://doi.org/10.1027/1192-5604/a000148

Meyer, G. J., & Friston, K. J. (2022). The active Bayesian brain and the Rorschach task. *Rorschachiana, 43*(2), 128–150. https://doi.org/10.1027/1192-5604/a000158

Meyer, G. J., Viglione, D. J., Mihura, J. L., Erard, R. E., & Erdberg, P. (2011). *Rorschach Performance Assessment System: Administration, coding, interpretation, and technical manual.* Rorschach Performance Assessment System.

Meyer, G. J., Giromini, L., Viglione, D. J., Reese, J. B., & Mihura, J. L. (2015). The association of gender, ethnicity, age, and education with Rorschach scores. *Assessment, 22*(1), 46–64. https://doi.org/10.1177/1073191114544358

O'Neill, R. M. (2005). Body image, body boundary, and the Barrier and Penetration Rorschach Scoring System. In R. F. Bornstein & J. M. Masling (Eds.), *Scoring the Rorschach: Seven validated systems* (pp. 159–189). Lawrence Erlbaum Associates Publishers.

Rorschach, H. (1921). *Psychodiagnostik: Methodik und Ergebnisse eines Warhrnehmungs-diagnostischen Experiments (Deutenlassen von Zufallsformen)* [Psychodiagnostics: Methodology and results of a perception-diagnostic experiment (interpretation of random forms)]. E. Bircher.

Rorschach, H. (2021). *Hermann Rorschach's psychodiagnostics: Newly translated and annotated 100th anniversary edition* (P. J. Keddy, R. Signer, P. Erdberg, & A. Schneider-Stocking, Trans. & Eds.). Hogrefe Publishing. (Original work published 1921)

Published online October 21, 2022

Filippo Aschieri
European Center for Therapeutic Assessment
Università Cattolica del Sacro Cuore
L.go Gemelli 1
2123 Milan
Italy
filippo.aschieri@unicatt.it

Invited Article

Toward an Integrative Perspective on the Person

Using Rorschach Data to Enhance the Diagnostic Systems

Robert F. Bornstein

Derner School of Psychology, Adelphi University, Garden City, NY, USA

Abstract: The *Diagnostic and Statistical Manual of Mental Disorders* (DSM) and *International Classification of Diseases* (ICD) have been criticized frequently in recent years, with most critiques focusing on perceived limitations of diagnostic categories. These criticisms notwithstanding, the most promising approach to refining the diagnostic systems is not to replace the categorical model, but to expand the range of assessment methods that are used by clinicians to render diagnoses. This article presents an evidence-based framework for integrating interview and Rorschach data to enhance diagnostic precision, improve treatment planning, and provide a novel paradigm for studying the dynamics of psychopathology in clinical and community settings. Following a discussion of problems associated with monomethod assessment based on patient self-reports, the advantages of multimethod assessment in psychiatric diagnosis are described. A three-step approach to evidence-based multimethod diagnosis is outlined, emphasizing patients' underlying dynamics, self-attributions, and expressed behaviors. The possibility of updating DSM and ICD symptom criteria to capture these three levels of patient functioning is discussed, strategies for exploring convergences and divergences between interview and Rorschach data are presented, and avenues for expanding the scope of Rorschach practice and research in the 21st century are described.

Keywords: Rorschach inkblot method, diagnostic interview, evidence-based diagnosis, multimethod assessment, process-focused model

How can we strengthen psychiatric diagnosis to obtain a more complete picture of the patient? The two dominant diagnostic systems in use today, the *Diagnostic and Statistical Manual of Mental Disorders* (DSM) and *International Classification of Diseases* (ICD), have been criticized frequently in recent years, with much of this criticism focusing on perceived limitations of categorical diagnoses (Hopwood et al., 2018; Krueger & Markon, 2014). Clinicians and clinical researchers have proposed replacing diagnostic categories with a series of dimensional ratings, arguing that a trait-based approach will be more heuristic and clinically useful than the current categorical model. Recent work in this area has focused primarily on personality disorders (PDs), but researchers have proposed applying a dimensional framework to symptom disorders as well, developing the influential

Hierarchical Taxonomy of Psychopathology (HiToP) to accomplish this goal (Kotov et al., 2017; Ruggero et al., 2019).

Although there are indeed some conceptual difficulties associated with certain DSM and ICD diagnoses, it is not clear that replacing these categories with a dimensional model will improve the reliability, validity, and clinical utility of contemporary diagnostic rubrics (Herpertz et al., 2017; Zachar & First, 2015). The most promising approach to refining psychiatric diagnoses is not to replace the categorical framework, but to expand the range of assessment methods that are used by clinicians to render diagnoses. By integrating information derived from diagnostic interviews with data from the Rorschach Inkblot Method (RIM), it may be possible to enhance diagnostic precision, improve treatment planning, and provide a novel paradigm for studying the dynamics of psychopathology in clinical and community settings. This article presents an evidence-based framework for using Rorschach data to enhance the diagnostic systems, focusing primarily on the assessment and diagnosis of PDs. Although the underlying dynamics associated with different PDs are particularly amenable to being assessed via the Rorschach, the framework presented here applies to other forms of psychopathology as well, including mood disorders, eating disorders, anxiety disorders, and thought disorders (see Bornstein, 2019b; Weiner & Kleiger, 2021).

An Unanswered Question and an Inconvenient Truth

With this as context, consider a disarmingly simple question, and one which many psychologists have not thought about very much: Why do the diagnostic manuals devote minimal attention to issues regarding assessment? The DSM and ICD both offer detailed guidelines regarding symptom criteria that must be met for a disorder to be diagnosed, but neither manual discusses how these criteria should be quantified. It is worth noting that unlike DSM and ICD, the current edition of the Psychodynamic Diagnostic Manual (PDM-2; Lingiardi & McWilliams, 2017) discusses assessment issues in considerable detail. It includes a separate chapter, 90 pages long, describing useful assessment strategies, along with recommendations for specific tests and measures, including the Rorschach, that capture key features of psychopathology, and other aspects of mental functioning.

To return to the question: Why have the DSM and ICD tended to neglect issues related to assessment? The primary reason for this is that both manuals implicitly equate the constructs they describe with the methods that are used to assess them. For example, in DSM-5-TR (American Psychiatric Association [APA], 2022), avoidant PD is diagnosed when a patient qualifies for 4 of 7 symptoms. It is assumed that the presence of these symptoms should be inferred based on information obtained in a diagnostic interview. In some instances, interview data may be supplemented and corroborated by archival evidence, or by the reports of knowledgeable informants. However, in the vast majority of situations, and in most clinical settings, diagnoses are based primarily on patient self-reports.

This approach has a long history, and if one looks back at the development of diagnostic criteria in DSM and ICD, taking a broad view, the process goes something like this. Early in the history of a syndrome, core symptoms are identified via clinical observation and research evidence. Once clinicians and clinical researchers are convinced that they understand the key symptoms of various disorders, clinical interviews are developed to quantify these symptoms. Sometimes questionnaire measures are developed as well, primarily to be used as screening tools. Studies are then conducted to document the reliability and validity of information obtained via these questionnaires and interviews, and once enough evidence has accumulated, practitioners render diagnoses based on data derived from these measures. Patients' reports of symptom-related phenomena are a primary source of evidence for the presence of psychological symptoms and disorders.

Monomethod Assessment and the "Illusion of Accuracy"

Relying on patients' self-reports to quantify symptom criteria is understandable, but it is problematic as well. It artificially inflates the perceived accuracy of information collected in a diagnostic interview. Meyer (2002) described this phenomenon as the "illusion of accuracy." In discussing the dynamics of this process, Meyer (2002, p. 78) noted:

> My main thesis here is that different sources of information provide distinct clinical data that are relevant to the diagnostic process. A hypothesis that flows from this is that as methods of information gathering become more distinct, the extent of association between different data sources will decline. Stated differently, to the extent that sources of information overlap or become confounded with each other, cross-source diagnostic agreement will become elevated. This can lead to an illusion of accuracy whereby a given source of diagnostic information is viewed as more accurate or trustworthy than is warranted.

The illusion of accuracy that Meyer (2002) describes not only makes interview data appear more valid than they really are, it also masks the fact that because questionnaire and interview-based studies of psychological disorders often use one form of self-report to predict another form of self-report, many of the conclusions that we draw regarding symptoms and diagnoses are less robust than they seem. This is true in clinical contexts, and in research settings as well (Bornstein, 2003, 2011b).

What do DSM and ICD Symptom Criteria Really Measure?

The problems associated with monomethod assessment notwithstanding, a skeptic might argue that there is no need to go beyond interview data in rendering diagnoses because the diagnostic manuals have evolved to the point that symptom criteria are now largely behavioral, or at any rate, observable. Underlying dynamics are mentioned less frequently in recent editions of the DSM and ICD than had been the case in earlier versions of these manuals. The question remains: What proportion of PD symptoms in recent editions of the diagnostic manuals tap underlying dynamics rather than expressed behaviors?

To address this issue Bornstein et al. (2014) classified the 92 PD symptoms in DSM-5 (APA, 2013) into four categories based on the domains of impairment in the manual's *General Diagnostic Criteria for a Personality Disorder*: cognition, affectivity, interpersonal functioning, and impulse control. Bornstein et al. found that the most common form of impairment for DSM-5 PDs is interpersonal functioning, which comprises 41% of all PD symptoms. This is followed by cognition (30%), and affectivity (18%), with relatively few symptoms (6%) reflecting difficulties in impulse control. Most important in the present context, about half of the DSM-5 PD symptoms, 48%, describe internal mental states – thought patterns and emotional responses. Similar percentages characterize PD symptom criteria in the ICD-10 (World Health Organization [WHO], 1994). As a result, in most clinical settings diagnosticians have relied on patient self-reports to document problematic thoughts and emotions as well as maladaptive behavior patterns. There are at least three difficulties with this approach.

First, self-reports of psychological symptoms are influenced by patients' symptom-related schemas, language constraints, and expectations regarding "normal" behavior. Cultural confounds pervade these self-reports, as do confounds related to patient gender, age, and other variables. As Wilson and Dunn (2004, p. 493) noted, part of the problem lies in the architecture of the human mental apparatus, because a fair amount of information about one's internal states simply cannot be accessed directly. In their words,

A common source of self-knowledge failure is the inaccessibility of much of the mind to consciousness, including mental processes involved in perception, motor learning, personality, attitudes, and self-esteem. Introspection cannot provide a direct pipeline to these mental processes, though some types of introspection may help people construct beneficial personal narratives.

A second source of bias comes from the diagnostician. All clinicians – even those who work hard to overcome their preconceptions and stereotypes – make implicit assumptions regarding patients based on characteristics such as their gender, ethnicity, socioeconomic status, sexuality, and age (Croskerry et al., 2013). It is very difficult to attenuate these reflexive responses, and they compromise diagnostic accuracy in myriad ways. Studies confirm that clinicians begin to draw conclusions regarding patients based on just a few moments of interaction, and then, without realizing it, they engage in "self-fulfilling interviewing" – a form of confirmatory bias. Diagnosticians tend to ask questions that support their initial conclusions, and fail to consider diagnoses that conflict with their initial gut reaction.

Beyond the separate biases of patient and therapist, some distortions are rooted in the patient-therapist interaction. All clinical interviews, including diagnostic interviews, are dialogues wherein patient and therapist create meaning out of ambiguity (Wilshire et al., 2021). Symptoms and diagnoses are co-constructed by patient and therapist. So are causal factors presumed to underlie symptoms. As the interview proceeds, therapist and patient gradually develop a shared consensus regarding the nature of the patient's difficulties. The "beneficial personal narratives" described by Wilson and Dunn (2004) are not constructed solely by the patient; the diagnostician co-authors these narratives as well.

Advantages of Combining Self-Reports and Rorschach Data

There is no way to eliminate completely those biases that stem from the patient, the diagnostician, and the patient–diagnostician interaction. The best that one can do is to identify them, and take steps to minimize them. Use of multimethod assessment, combining interview and Rorschach data to inform diagnosis, will go a long way toward meeting that goal. Multimethod assessment is particularly important for accurate diagnosis of personality pathology, where patient self-reports are notoriously inaccurate (Huprich et al., 2011), but it is true of many other types of pathology as well (Weiner & Kleiger, 2021).

Bornstein's (1998) study examining the patterns of underlying and expressed dependency needs in dependent and histrionic PDs confirms the clinical and heuristic value of multimethod assessment in this context. To address the long-standing clinical hypothesis that unconscious dependency strivings may play a role in histrionic pathology, this study assessed underlying and self-reported dependency needs in two groups of college students, one of whom met DSM-IV (APA, 1994) criteria for histrionic PD, and the other of whom met the criteria for dependent PD. All participants completed a self-report measure of dependency, the Interpersonal Dependency Inventory (Hirschfeld et al., 1977), as well as the Rorschach Oral Dependency scale (Bornstein & Masling, 2005), which is now formalized as the Oral Dependent Language scale in the Rorschach Performance Assessment System (R-PAS; Meyer et al., 2011), and has been included as a Supplementary Scale in the Comprehensive System (CS; Smith et al., 2022). As expected, participants in the dependent PD group showed high levels of both underlying and self-reported dependency, whereas those in the histrionic PD group scored high on underlying dependency, but not self-reported dependency. Figure 1 illustrates the patterns of underlying and expressed dependency needs in these two groups of participants, with histrionic participants' test scores placing them primarily in the lower left portion of Figure 1 ("Unacknowledged Dependency"), and dependent participants' test scores placing them in the lower right portion of this figure ("High Dependency").

Bornstein's (1998) study provided the first direct evidence that dependent PD is associated with high levels of both underlying and expressed dependency, whereas histrionic PD is associated with high levels of underlying dependency, but not self-reported dependency. This study and its findings actually altered the description of histrionic personality disorder in DSM-IV-TR (APA, 2000) and DSM-5 (APA, 2013), where, for the first time, the role of underlying dependency strivings in histrionicity was noted. In describing the dynamics of histrionic patients, the DSM-5 stated that "They may seek to control their partner through emotional manipulation or seductiveness on one level, while displaying a marked dependency on them at another level" (APA, 2013, p. 668). These results provide a noteworthy example of how Rorschach findings helped refine a DSM diagnosis. There are many more areas where this can, and should, occur.

Multimethod Assessment and Evidence-Based Diagnosis

Given the limitations of diagnoses based exclusively on interview data, multimethod assessment should be considered a key element – a defining feature – of evidence-based diagnosis. Although there is a wealth of writing on evidence-based treatment (Spring, 2007), and evidence-based assessment (Bornstein, 2017), there is only a modest amount of writing on evidence-based diagnosis.

SCORE ON
SELF-REPORT DEPENDENCY TEST

		LOW	HIGH
SCORE ON PERFORMANCE BASED DEPENDENCY TEST	LOW	Low Implicit Low Self-Attributed **Low Dependency**	Low Implicit High Self-Attributed **Dependent Self-Presentation**
	HIGH	High Implicit Low Self-Attributed **Unacknowledged Dependency**	High Implicit High Self-Attributed **High Dependency**

Figure 1. Continuities and discontinuities in implicit and self-attributed dependency test scores. The upper left and lower right panels reflect convergences between implicit and self-attributed dependency strivings; the lower left and upper right panels illustrate discontinuities. The lower left cell includes those patients who appear to have high levels of underlying dependency but are unaware of this, or unwilling to acknowledge it when asked. The upper right cell includes patients who appear to have low levels of implicit dependency needs but nonetheless choose to present themselves as being highly dependent. Reprinted with permission from the *Annual Review of Clinical Psychology*, Volume 8, by Annual Reviews, http://www.annualreviews.org.

That which exists does not address the value of combining self-reports with measures like the Rorschach (see, e.g., Youngstrom et al., 2015).

To combine interview and Rorschach data effectively in diagnostic settings, it is important to have a clear understanding of the psychological processes engaged by these two assessment tools. Bornstein's (2011b) process-focused classification of psychological tests, which organizes measures into six categories based on the processes engaged by each measure, provides a useful framework for addressing this issue.

From a process-focused perspective, clinical interviews tap two things. First and foremost, they emphasize patients' descriptions of their expressed behaviors and internal mental states. In that respect interviews are like "verbal questionnaires." Beyond the patient's verbalizations, however, the clinician's observations and inferences also play a role in determining the conclusions that emerge during diagnostic interviews (Sommers-Flanagan, 2016). Regardless of how a patient may describe their thought processes, if the diagnostician observes cognitive slippage and loosening of associations during the interview, that information will help shape the clinician's conclusions. Regardless of how a patient perceives and describes their emotional patterns, if that patient becomes dysregulated during the interview, the clinician will take this into account when rendering a diagnosis.

The Rorschach taps a very different set of psychological processes. Here the patient is not asked to describe themselves, but to attribute meaning to an ambiguous stimulus, with these attributions determined in part by stimulus characteristics, and in part by the person's cognitive style, motives, emotions, and need states (see Exner, 2003; Meyer et al., 2011). Over the years the Rorschach has been described as a projective test, free-response test, and performance-based test, but "stimulus-attribution test" is really a more accurate label. The meaning we ascribe to inkblots is the end result of an attribution process, except that in contrast to questionnaires and interviews, where the patient is asked to generate a series of self-attributions, here they are asked to attribute meaning to external stimuli: stimulus attributions.

Combining Interview and Rorschach Data to Enhance Diagnosis

Understanding the psychological processes that underlie interview and Rorschach responses is important, but it is also necessary to have a framework that will enable clinicians to synthesize relevant information, and integrate these contrasting sources of data to obtain as complete a picture as possible of the person. Three steps are involved.

Step 1: Identify the Underlying Dynamics, Expressed Behaviors, and Self-Attributions Associated With a Particular Disorder

As with any evidence-based framework, it is crucial to begin with the published literature – research studies and clinical writings. Using this literature, we can articulate the underlying dynamics, expressed behaviors, and self-attributions that characterize a given syndrome. In other words, in describing and diagnosing a psychological disorder, the clinician is asking three distinct questions. First, what are the most important psychological dynamics associated with that disorder – the motives, urges, conflicts, defenses, coping strategies, and emotional patterns experienced by the patient, some of which may not be fully accessible to conscious awareness. Second, what sorts of self-attributions would we expect a patient with this disorder to make: How do they perceive themselves, and how do they describe themselves when asked? Third, what patterns of behavior would we expect a patient with this type of psychopathology to display? How will they behave in everyday life, and how will they behave during the interview?

Step 2: Assess Patient Functioning in all Three Domains

Having developed a set of working hypotheses regarding the patient's underlying dynamics, self-attributions, and expressed behaviors, the diagnostician should assess patient functioning in these domains. Rorschach data will be particularly useful for assessing the underlying dynamics associated with a particular form of psychopathology. Interviews will be a particularly good source of information regarding the patient's self-attributions and behavior patterns.

Step 3: Interpret Assessment Results, With Attention to Cross-Method Convergences and Divergences

The final task in evidence-based multimethod diagnosis is to combine these data – to interpret the assessment results obtained in Step 2. Three guidelines are helpful here.

First, *contextualize*: Always interpret these data with reference to the psychological processes that were engaged when a particular piece of information was collected. In other words, whenever the clinician is trying to understand the implications of diagnostic information, they must ask: Is that information related to underlying dynamics, self-attributions, or expressed behavior?

Second, *integrate*: Seek areas of convergence between different sources of information – areas where evidence collected using different methods leads to similar conclusions. Sometimes Rorschach data are consistent with a patient's self-reports of emotional patterns or coping strategies. If so, this suggests that the patient has some degree of insight into these aspects of their functioning; knowing this is helpful in treatment planning.

Third, *contrast*: Seek areas of divergence between different sources of information – areas where evidence collected via different methods yields inconsistent results. There are numerous examples in the Rorschach literature of situations where divergences between Rorschach and self-report data tell us something important about individual patients (de Villemor-Amaral & Finn, 2020; Fondren & Jenkins, 2020; Husain, 2015; Keddy & Erdberg, 2010). There are also numerous examples of situations where these divergences inform us about psychological dynamics more broadly (Berant et al., 2008; Cogswell et al., 2010; Van Laer et al., 2020). These discontinuities are central to evidence-based diagnosis in clinical settings, and analyzing these cross-method discrepancies is important in forensic contexts as well (Erard & Evans, 2017; Mihura, 2012).

Combining Interview and Rorschach Data to Illuminate Maladaptive Dependency

To illustrate how this process might play itself out as the clinician integrates interview and Rorschach data to capture the underlying dynamics, self-attributions, and expressed behaviors that characterize a specific form of personality pathology, consider a hypothetical patient who presents with dysfunctional, maladaptive dependency. How might this dependent patient describe themself during a diagnostic interview? In other words, what is their characteristic pattern of self-attributions? We know that when asked, dependent people typically describe themselves as being insecure, anxious, and needy. Dependent people generally describe themselves as being accommodating and compliant as well, willing to go along with what others want, and put others' needs before their own to avoid disrupting the relationship (Bornstein, 2006).

When we compare dependent patients' self-attributions with their characteristic patterns of behavior, it becomes clear that these self-attributions do not reflect what most dependent patients actually do in the real world. Dependent people may describe themselves as being acquiescent and accommodating, but their behavior is quite variable depending upon the contingencies that characterize different situations. Some dependent patients tend to be relatively passive, others more assertive, but all exhibit an array of social influence strategies ranging from passive to active, depending upon the circumstances (see Bornstein, 2011a, 2012, for a review of research in this area). Some dependent people can be quite aggressive when they perceive important relationships to be at risk (Bornstein, 2019a; Bornstein & O'Neill, 2000).

We also have a good idea of how dependent people perform on the Rorschach, and other stimulus-attribution tests. Decades of research confirms that they tend to report a high proportion of oral dependent imagery (Aschieri et al., 2021; Bornstein & Masling, 2005; Meyer et al., 2011; Smith et al., 2022). They produce a higher-than-average number of dependent percepts – images of figures that are vulnerable or helpless, and in need of external support. They also produce high numbers of food- and mouth-related percepts.

Beyond the Rorschach Oral Dependency (ROD) Scale, and the Oral Dependent Language (ODL) Scale, there are certain Rorschach variables that can be very informative in capturing the underlying dynamics associated with a particular patient's dependency. For example, when elevated ROD and ODL scores are coupled with a high number of structural special scores – boundary violations – it may suggest the presence of borderline pathology (Bornstein et al., 2010). Conversely, when elevated ROD and ODL scores are accompanied by a positive Mutuality of

Autonomy index, or Cooperative Movement score, the diagnostician can entertain the possibility that this patient expresses underlying dependency strivings in relatively adaptive ways (see Denckla et al., 2015; Huprich et al., 2013, for evidence regarding healthy versus unhealthy expressions of underlying dependency). Either of these patterns would have important implications for treatment planning and risk management.

Updating Diagnostic Rubrics to Capture Multiple Levels of Functioning

Scrutiny of this description of the hypothetical dependent patient's underlying dynamics, self-attributions, and expressed behaviors raises an important issue: These aspects of pathological dependency are not formalized in the diagnostic manuals. They are not captured in DSM and ICD symptom criteria for dependent PD. Moreover, this limitation is not unique to dependent PD, but represents a significant problem that affects a large number of diagnostic categories. There is a disconnect between what we know are the most important elements of certain forms of psychopathology, and what is included in the DSM and ICD symptom lists (Livesley, 2010; Yager & McIntyre, 2014).

Implementing evidence-based multi-method diagnosis in clinical settings requires a different approach on the part of the diagnostician, but changes may be needed in the diagnostic systems as well. Moving forward, it will be important that our diagnostic rubrics evolve to incorporate all three dimensions of patient functioning. Equally important, we should be clear regarding which dimension of functioning each symptom taps. In future versions of the diagnostic manuals each symptom should be explicitly identified according to the level of functioning that is captured by that symptom: underlying dynamics, self-attributions, or expressed behaviors.

Figure 2 presents a modified set of symptom criteria for dependent PD that is consistent with clinical and empirical evidence in this area, and captures all three elements of patient functioning. These diagnostic criteria begin, as the DSM-5-TR (APA, 2022) now does, with an overview of the disorder's essential features. Then, to maximize clinical utility, some symptoms tap the underlying dynamics associated with problematic dependency. Central to these dynamics is a perception of oneself as vulnerable and weak, coupled with a belief that other people are competent, confident, and strong. Dependent people also experience a strong desire to obtain and maintain stable attachments with potential caregivers, and anxiety regarding abandonment and relationship disruption (Bornstein, 2011a, 2012).

Dependent Personality Disorder

A view of the self as helpless and ineffectual that motivates the person to seek nurturant, protective relationships and exhibit an array of passive and active behaviors to maintain those relationships. This pattern is present in a variety of contexts, with severity of pathological dependency reflected in the degree of distress and impairment associated with the person's dependent beliefs, motives, and behaviors.

Underlying Dynamics

1) Perception of self as vulnerable and weak
2) Belief that other people are comparatively competent, confident, and strong
3) Strong desire to obtain and maintain stable attachments to potential caregivers
4) Anxiety regarding abandonment and relationship disruption

Self-Attributions

5) Self as accommodating, cooperative, flexible, and other-focused

Expressed Behaviors

6) Broad array of social influence strategies designed to strengthen ties to caregivers
7) Use of active as well as passive behaviors to preclude abandonment, including supplication, ingratiation, exemplification, and intimidation

---

Figure 2. Evidence-based diagnostic criteria for dependent PD.

How do dependent people describe themselves when asked? The characteristic self-attributions associated with high levels of interpersonal dependency include a perception of oneself as accommodating, cooperative, flexible, and other-focused (Bockian, 2009). The key issue here is to conceptualize these as what they are – self-attributions – rather than erroneously assuming they are accurate depictions of how the dependent person actually behaves.

Third, it is important to include symptoms that tap the patterns of expressed behavior exhibited by patients with high levels of underlying dependency. These include a broad array of social influence strategies ranging from supplication and ingratiation to exemplification and intimidation (Bornstein, 2006, 2019a). The diagnostician should note which social influence strategies are characteristic of a particular dependent patient's most important relationships, and how these social influence strategies vary across contexts and settings.

To provide another example, Figure 3 presents a process-focused set of symptom criteria for narcissistic PD, as might appear in a future version of DSM or ICD. Again, these criteria begin with the disorder's essential features. As Figure 3 shows, the core underlying dynamic in pathological narcissism is a view of oneself

---

Narcissistic Personality Disorder

A pervasive pattern of grandiosity, need for admiration, and lack of empathy; this pattern represents a form of overcompensation designed to keep underlying feelings of worthlessness outside conscious awareness. When defenses are effective in keeping these feelings from reaching consciousness grandiose narcissism results; when defenses are less effective vulnerable narcissism ensues.

Underlying Dynamics

1) Unconscious view of self as insignificant, unimportant, unloved, and unlovable
2) Hypersensitivity to evidence of personal weakness and vulnerability
3) Reliance on defenses such as denial and reaction formation to prevent troubling beliefs regarding the self from reaching conscious awareness

Self-Attributions

4) Self as important, valued, admired, respected, and deserving of special treatment

Expressed Behaviors

5) Grandiosity, egocentricity, and mistreatment of others perceived as being of lower status
6) Submissive, sycophantic behavior in the presence of those perceived as being more powerful

Figure 3. Evidence-based diagnostic criteria for narcissistic PD.

as insignificant and ineffectual, coupled with reliance on defenses such as denial and reaction formation which prevent these troubling beliefs from reaching conscious awareness (Zeigler-Hill et al., 2010). Evidence confirms that narcissistic people are actually hypersensitive to evidence of their own perceived weakness and vulnerability; they unconsciously seek out this evidence so they can ward it off and protect their fragile self-concept (Horvath & Morf, 2009; Morf et al., 2011).

Beyond these dynamics, narcissistic people show a characteristic set of self-attributions. They describe themselves as important, valued, admired, respected, and deserving of special treatment (Pincus & Lukowitsky, 2010; Ronningstam, 2011). Needless to say, these self-attributions do not reflect the underlying dynamics of narcissism – those thoughts, feelings, and fears that are so painful to the narcissistic patient – which is why it is important to keep these two things separate.

As is often these case with personality pathology, the narcissistic person's self-attributions also do not capture their expressed behaviors, which vary according to the perceived status of those around them. Narcissistic people do indeed display grandiosity, self-centeredness, and a tendency to mistreat others who are perceived as being of lower status. They then shift to submissive, even sycophantic behavior in the presence of those they perceive as being more powerful (Morf & Rhodewalt, 2001).

A Paradigm Shift in Personality Disorder Diagnosis

A proponent of the emerging dimensional PD model might argue that this three-tiered approach to multi-method diagnosis is interesting, but that dependency and narcissism are historical artifacts, soon to be removed altogether from the diagnostic manuals. We are in the midst of a paradigm shift in the conceptualization of personality pathology.

There is no doubt that the mental health professions are currently transitioning to a more dimensional, trait-focused framework for capturing normal and pathological functioning, but it is important to consider this shift within its broader historical context. No matter how compelling the dimensional framework may seem, this is not a permanent change in the way that personality pathology will be conceptualized and diagnosed. It is part of an ongoing dialectic that has been in place for more than a century (Bornstein, 2019b; Herpertz et al., 2017; Millon, 2011). Figure 4 illustrates the dynamics of this trait-type dialectic. As this figure shows, at certain times the pendulum swings in one direction, sometimes in the other. The pendulum is currently swinging from type to trait. Eventually it will swing back from trait to type (see Bornstein, 2019b, for a discussion of this dynamic; Lilienfeld, 2019 and Widiger, 2019, for contrasting perspectives).

Regardless of what the long-term future may hold, in ICD-11 (WHO, 2019) – and presumably in subsequent editions of the manual – PDs will be diagnosed using a series of trait ratings. HiToP (Kotov et al., 2017; Ruggero et al., 2019) extends this perspective to symptom disorders as well, articulating an integrative framework for conceptualizing and diagnosing a broad array of psychological syndromes – symptom disorders as well as PDs – from a dimensional perspective. Is multimethod diagnosis combining interview and Rorschach data useful when trait-focused frameworks are used?

The answer to this question is yes, because self-reports are also the predominant method for assessing trait domains and facets, though when traits are assessed, those self-reports typically take the form of questionnaire rather than interview responses (Krueger & Markon, 2014; Widiger, 2019). This creates assessment problems when patients are asked to describe feelings, motives, conflicts, and defenses about which they have may limited awareness. The same assessment challenges and opportunities that characterize categorical diagnostic rubrics characterize dimensional diagnostic frameworks. The same assessment tautology that

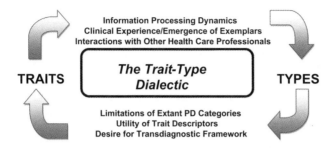

Figure 4. The trait–type dialectic. Intra- and interpersonal factors that favor traits over types are in the top portion of the figure; those that favor types over traits are in the bottom portion. © 2019 by the American Psychological Association. Reproduced with permission. Bornstein, R. F. (2019). The trait-type dialectic: Construct validity, clinical utility, and the diagnostic process. *Personality Disorders: Theory, Research, and Treatment*, *10*(3), 199–209.

limits the DSM's current symptom-focused model constrains trait-based models as well. The content of constructs being assessed may differ, but the process remains the same.

When we scrutinize the various features that comprise the ICD-11 (WHO, 2019) trait dimension of negative affectivity (e.g., anxiety, shame, low self-esteem), it becomes clear that many of these constructs are amenable to being assessed via the Rorschach. The same is true of the ICD-11 trait dimension of disinhibition, which includes the facets of impulsivity, distractibility, and lack of planning. As is true when symptom-focused diagnoses are rendered, the self-attributions that patients make when asked to describe their traits and behavioral predispositions are only modestly related to their actual expressed behavior (Bornstein, 2017; Meyer et al., 2001). Thus, evidence-based multimethod diagnosis enables researchers to integrate and contrast the key elements of trait-based models of psychopathology using the same logic, and same assessment strategies, as are used when diagnoses are rendered within the context of a categorical diagnostic system.

Moving Forward: An Agenda for the 21st Century

One hundred years ago, Hermann Rorschach undertook a "research experiment" (Rorschach, 1921) that eventually became something far more influential than he ever could have imagined. The RIM had modest beginnings, but over time the method began to reveal its power as a way of identifying aspects of personality and psychopathology that cannot be accessed via self-report. Decades of research have shown that the Rorschach is a powerful assessment tool which yields unique information that cannot be obtained via other methods (Hiller et al., 1999; Mihura et al., 2013). It has an evidence base that is comparable to – sometimes stronger than – the evidence base associated with other well-established testing procedures (see, e.g., Aschieri & Pascarella, 2021, for a review of evidence regarding changes in RIM scores during the course of psychotherapy, and Giromini et al., 2022, for the application of experimental procedures to examine the psychological processes underlying Rorschach responses).

Despite the Rorschach's many strengths, the orchestrated attacks on the RIM which took place in the 1990s and early 2000s had an impact on the Rorschach community that persists to this day. Rorschach researchers became so preoccupied with these criticisms that the perceived limitations of the RIM came to define the parameters of the debate. In response to these criticisms, researchers began to focus on demonstrating that the Rorschach was not flawed – that it was an adequate measure with acceptable psychometric properties.

It is time for the Rorschach community to reorient its goals, and set the bar higher. As we shepherd Rorschach's "research experiment" through its second century, it is time to put earlier misguided criticisms to rest and move forward. Two innovations can help maximize the clinical utility and heuristic value of the Rorschach within the diagnostic systems, and beyond them as well.

The Rorschach as Transdiagnostic Tool

The Oxford Language Dictionary Online defines the term *symptom* as "a physical or mental feature which is regarded as indicating a condition of disease" (https://languages.oup.com/research/oxford-english-dictionary). With this definition in mind, we can strengthen future versions of the diagnostic rubrics by expanding our understanding of what constitutes a symptom of psychological disorder. It would enhance diagnostic precision if we formally conceptualize Rorschach patterns that are highly predictive of a particular syndrome as "symptoms", just as we do with patients' interview-derived self-attributions and behavior patterns. If direct verbalizations (interview-based self-reports) represent *prima facie* evidence of psychopathology, why should indirect verbalizations (Rorschach patterns) not represent similar evidence?

Viewed through this lens, the Rorschach has the potential to become a transdiagnostic tool – a measure that can identify underlying dynamics common to different disorders and provide important information regarding overlap between ostensibly distinct syndromes. Borsboom et al. (2011) have made a compelling argument that symptoms shared by multiple disorders – what they call "bridge symptoms" – tell us a great deal about the structure of psychopathology, and the relationships among different disorders (see also Borsboom & Cramer, 2013). The same may be true regarding shared Rorschach patterns. If high M-% coupled with low Cooperative Movement is a pattern common to two or more forms of psychopathology, perhaps that tells us something important about an overlapping dynamic that characterizes those two syndromes.

Enhancing the Research Domain Criteria

About 10 years ago policymakers at the National Institute of Mental Health in the United States developed the Research Domain Criteria, a framework articulating various levels of analysis that are useful for studying the psychological processes which underlie healthy and disordered functioning (Stoyanov et al., 2019). These criteria – now commonly referred to as RDoC – tend to emphasize the physiological underpinnings of various mental processes, and prioritize evidence bearing on genetics, neural circuitry, and other physiological indices (e.g., heart rate, cortisol levels; see Cuthbert, 2022). What most clinicians think of as the more traditional forms of psychological test data – self-reports and behavioral assessments – represent a small portion of the RDoC assessment framework.

RDoC's emphases notwithstanding, decades of research and clinical experience confirm that performance-based testing yields unique information that is conceptually and methodologically distinct from the information provided via self-reports and expressed behaviors. By examining convergences and divergences between performance-based test data and data obtained using these other two assessment methods, we obtain a more nuanced perspective regarding a person's psychological functioning. Performance-based test data should be included in RDoC as a separate level of analysis, alongside behavior and self-report. The Rorschach community is ideally situated to integrate performance-based testing into RDoC, setting the stage for continued interest in the RIM among clinicians, and among researchers as well.

Conclusion

The Rorschach is a uniquely powerful measure of underlying psychological dynamics, adding incremental validity (i.e., unique predictive value) in diagnostic settings, and complementing self-report data to provide a more complete picture of the patient. The framework described here not only has the potential to enhance psychiatric diagnosis and improve treatment planning, but this framework can enable the RIM to play a central role in evidence-based diagnosis and assessment in a variety of contexts and settings. Because many assessment procedures involve integrating evidence from measures that draw upon a diverse array of psychological processes (e.g., assessment of intelligence, competency, vocational aptitude, and neuropsychological functioning), the principles outlined here may be useful in refining these tasks as well.

References

American Psychiatric Association. (1994). *Diagnostic and statistical manual of mental disorders* (4th ed.).

American Psychiatric Association. (2000). *Diagnostic and statistical manual of mental disorders* (4th ed., text rev.).

American Psychiatric Association. (2013). *Diagnostic and statistical manual of mental disorders* (5th ed.).

American Psychiatric Association. (2022). *Diagnostic and statistical manual of mental disorders* (5th ed., text rev.).

Aschieri, F., Brusadelli, E., Durosini, I., Tomasich, A., & Giromini, L. (2021). Cross-cultural applicability of Oral–Dependent Language (ODL). *Professional Psychology: Research and Practice, 52*(5), 461–469. https://doi.org/10.1037/pro0000343

Aschieri, F., & Pascarella, G. (2021). A systematic narrative review of evaluating change in psychotherapy with the Rorschach Test. *Rorschachiana, 42*(2), 232–257. https://doi.org/10.1027/1192-5604/a000142

Berant, E., Newborn, M., & Orgler, S. (2008). Convergence of self-report scales and Rorschach indexes of psychological distress: The moderating role of self-disclosure. *Journal of Personality Assessment, 90*(1), 36–43. https://doi.org/10.1080/00223890701693702

Bockian, N. (2009). *Personality-guided therapy for depression.* APA Books.

Bornstein, R. F. (1998). Implicit and self-attributed dependency needs in dependent and histrionic personality disorders. *Journal of Personality Assessment, 71*(1), 1–14. https://doi.org/10.1207/s15327752jpa7101_1

Bornstein, R. F. (2003). Behaviorally referenced experimentation and symptom validation: A paradigm for 21st century personality disorder research. *Journal of Personality Disorders, 17*(1), 1–18. https://doi.org/10.1521/pedi.17.1.1.24056

Bornstein, R. F. (2006). The complex relationship between dependency and domestic violence: Converging psychological factors and social forces. *American Psychologist, 61*(6), 595–606. https://doi.org/10.1037/0003-066X.61.6.595

Bornstein, R. F. (2011a). An interactionist perspective on interpersonal dependency. *Current Directions in Psychological Science, 20*(2), 124–128. https://doi.org/10.1177/0963721411403121

Bornstein, R. F. (2011b). Toward a process-focused model of test score validity: Improving psychological assessment in science and practice. *Psychological Assessment, 23*(2), 532–544. https://doi.org/10.1037/a0022402

Bornstein, R. F. (2012). From dysfunction to adaptation: An interactionist model of dependency. *Annual Review of Clinical Psychology, 8*, 291–316. https://doi.org/10.1146/annurev-clinpsy-032511-143058

Bornstein, R. F. (2017). Evidence based psychological assessment. *Journal of Personality Assessment, 99*(4), 435–445. https://doi.org/10.1080/00223891.2016.1236343

Bornstein, R. F. (2019a). Synergistic dependencies in partner and elder abuse. *American Psychologist, 74*(6), 713–724. https://doi.org/10.1037/amp0000456

Bornstein, R. F. (2019b). The trait-type dialectic: Construct validity, clinical utility, and the diagnostic process. *Personality Disorders: Theory, Research, and Treatment, 10*(3), 199–209. https://doi.org/10.1037/per0000299

Bornstein, R. F., Becker-Matero, N., Winarick, D. J., & Reichman, A. E. (2010). Interpersonal dependency in borderline personality disorder: Clinical context and empirical evidence. *Journal of Personality Disorders, 24*(1), 109–127. https://doi.org/10.1521/pedi.2010.24.1.109

Bornstein, R. F., Bianucci, V., Fishman, D. P., & Biars, J. W. (2014). Toward a firmer foundation for DSM-5.1: Domains of impairment in DSM-IV/DSM-5 personality disorders. *Journal of Personality Disorders, 28*(2), 212–224. https://doi.org/10.1521/pedi_2013_27_116

Bornstein, R. F., & Masling, J. M. (2005). The Rorschach Oral Dependency Scale. In R. F. Bornstein & J. M. Masling (Eds.), *Scoring the Rorschach: Seven validated systems* (pp. 135–157). Erlbaum.

Bornstein, R. F., & O'Neill, R. M. (2000). Dependency and suicidality in psychiatric inpatients. *Journal of Clinical Psychology, 56*(4), 463–473. https://doi.org/10.1002/(SICI)1097-4679(200004)56:4<463::AID-JCLP2>3.0.CO;2-5

Borsboom, D., Cramer, A. O. J., Schmittmann, V. D., Epskamp, S., & Waldorp, L. J. (2011). The small world of psychopathology. *PLoS One, 6*(11), Article e27407. https://doi.org/10.1371/journal.pone.0027407

Borsboom, D., & Cramer, A. O. J. (2013). Network analysis: An integrative approach to the structure of psychopathology. *Annual Review of Clinical Psychology, 9*, 91–121. https://doi.org/10.1146/annurev-clinpsy-050212-185608

Cogswell, A., Alloy, L. B., Karpinski, A., & Grant, D. A. (2010). Assessing dependency using self-report and indirect measures: Examining the significance of discrepancies. *Journal of Personality Assessment, 92*(4), 306–316. https://doi.org/10.1080/00223891.2010.481986

Croskerry, P., Singhal, G., & Mamede, S. (2013). Cognitive debiasing 1: Origins of bias and theory of debiasing. *BMJ Quality and Safety, 22*, ii58–ii64. https://doi.org/10.1136/bmjqs-2013-002387

Cuthbert, B. N. (2022). Research Domain Criteria (RDoC): Progress and potential. *Current Directions in Psychological Science, 31*(2), 107–114. https://doi.org/10.1177/09637214211051363

Denckla, C. A., Bornstein, R. F., Mancini, A. D., & Bonanno, G. A. (2015). Disambiguating dependency and attachment among conjugally bereaved adults. *Journal of Loss and Trauma, 20*(5), 468–483. https://doi.org/10.1080/15325024.2014.949148

de Villemor-Amaral, A. E., & Finn, S. E. (2020). The Rorschach as a window into past traumas during therapeutic assessment. *Rorschachiana, 41*(2), 93–106. https://doi.org/10.1027/1192-5604/a000125

Erard, R. E. & Evans, F. B. (Eds.). (2017). *The Rorschach in multimethod forensic assessment*. Routledge/Taylor & Francis.

Exner, J. E. Jr. (2003). *The Rorschach: A comprehensive system* (4th ed.). John Wiley & Sons.

Fondren, A. H., & Jenkins, S. R. (2020). Horseshoe crabs and stingrays: A case study of interpersonal theory and multimethod collaborative/therapeutic assessment. *Rorschachiana, 41*(2), 162–180. https://doi.org/10.1027/1192-5604/a000129

Giromini, L., Lettieri, S. C., Bosi, J., & Zennaro, A. (2022). The effects of subliminal emotional priming on Rorschach responses. *Rorschachiana, 43*(1), 1–24. https://doi.org/10.1027/1192-5604/a000157

Herpertz, S. C., Huprich, S. K., Bohus, M., Chanen, A., Goodman, M., Mehlum, L., Moran, P., Newton-Howes, G., Scott, L., & Sharp, C. (2017). The challenge of transforming the diagnostic system of personality disorders. *Journal of Personality Disorders, 31*(5), 577–589. https://doi.org/10.1521/pedi_2017_31_338

Hiller, J. B., Rosenthal, R., Bornstein, R. F., Berry, D. T. R., & Brunell-Neulieb, S. (1999). A comparative meta-analysis of Rorschach and MMPI validity. *Psychological Assessment, 11*(3), 278–296. https://doi.org/10.1037/1040-3590.11.3.278

Hirschfeld, R. M. A., Klerman, G. L., Gough, H. G., Barrett, J., Korchin, S. J., & Chodoff, P. (1977). A measure of interpersonal dependency. *Journal of Personality Assessment, 41*(6), 610–618. https://doi.org/10.1207/s15327752jpa4106_6

Hopwood, C. J., Kotov, R., Krueger, R. F., Watson, D., Widiger, T. A., Althoff, R. R., Ansell, E. B., Bach, B., Bagby, R. M., Blais, M. A., Bornovalova, M. A., Chmielewski, M., Cicero, D. C., Conway, C., De Clercq, B., De Fruyt, F., Docherty, A. R., Eaton, N. R., Edens, J. F., ... Zimmermann, J. (2018). The time has come for dimensional personality disorder diagnosis. *Personality and Mental Health, 12*(1), 82–86. https://doi.org/10.1002/pmh.1408

Horvath, S., & Morf, C. C. (2009). Narcissistic defensiveness: Hypervigilance and avoidance of worthlessness. *Journal of Experimental Social Psychology, 45*(6), 1252–1258. https://doi.org/10.1016/j.jesp.2009.07.011

Huprich, S. K., Bornstein, R. F., & Schmitt, T. A. (2011). Self-report methodology is insufficient for improving the assessment and classification of Axis II personality disorders. *Journal of Personality Disorders, 25*(5), 557–570. https://doi.org/10.1521/pedi.2011.25.5.557

Huprich, S. K., Hoban, P., Boys, A., & Rosen, A. (2013). Healthy and maladaptive dependency and its relationship to pain management and perceptions in physical therapy patients. *Journal of Clinical Psychology in Medical Settings, 20*(4), 508–514. https://doi.org/10.1007/s10880-013-9372-1

Husain, O. (2015). From persecution to depression: A case of chronic depression – Associating the Rorschach, the TAT, and Winnicott. *Journal of Personality Assessment, 97*(3), 230–240. https://doi.org/10.1080/00223891.2015.1009081

Keddy, P., & Erdberg, P. (2010). Changes in the Rorschach and MMPI-2 after electroconvulsive therapy (ECT): A collaborative assessment case study. *Journal of Personality Assessment, 92*(4), 279–295. https://doi.org/10.1080/00223891.2010.481982

Kotov, R., Krueger, R. F., Watson, D., Achenbach, T. M., Althoff, R. R., Bagby, R. M., Brown, T. A., Carpenter, W. T., Caspi, A., Clark, L. A., Eaton, N. R., Forbes, M. K., Forbush, K. T., Goldberg, D., Hasin, D., Hyman, S. E., Ivanova, M. Y., Lynam, D. R., Markon, K., ... Zimmerman, M. (2017). The Hierarchical Taxonomy of Psychopathology (HiTOP): A dimensional alternative to traditional nosologies. *Journal of Abnormal Psychology, 126*(4), 454–477. https://doi.org/10.1037/abn0000258

Krueger, R. F., & Markon, K. E. (2014). The role of the DSM-5 personality trait model in moving toward a quantitative and empirically based approach to classifying personality and psychopathology. *Annual Review of Clinical Psychology, 10*, 477–501. https://doi.org/10.1146/annurev-clinpsy-032813-153732

Lingiardi, V. & McWilliams, N. (Eds.). (2017). *Psychodynamic diagnostic manual: PDM-2* (2nd ed.). The Guilford Press.

Lilienfeld, S. O. (2019). Reflections on clinical judgment and the dimensional–categorical distinction in the study of personality disorders: Comment on Bornstein (2019). *Personality Disorders: Theory, Research, and Treatment, 10*(3), 210–214. https://doi.org/10.1037/per0000318

Livesley, W. J. (2010). Confusion and incoherence in the classification of personality disorder: Commentary on the preliminary proposals for DSM-5. *Psychological Injury and Law, 3*(4), 304–313. https://doi.org/10.1007/s12207-010-9094-8

Meyer, G. J. (2002). Implications of information-gathering methods for a refined taxonomy of psychopathology. In L. E. Beutler & M. L. Malik (Eds.), *Rethinking the DSM: A psychological perspective* (pp. 69–105). American Psychological Association.

Meyer, G. J., Finn, S. E., Eyde, L. D., Kay, G. G., Moreland, K. L., Dies, R. R., Eisman, E. J., Kubiszyn, T. W., & Reed, G. M. (2001). Psychological testing and psychological assessment: A review of evidence and issues. *American Psychologist, 56*(2), 128–165. https://doi.org/10.1037/0003-066X.56.2.128

Meyer, G. J., Viglione, D. J., Mihura, J. L., Erard, R. E., & Erdberg, P. (2011). *Rorschach performance assessment system: Administration, coding, interpretation and technical manual*. Rorschach Performance Assessment System.

Mihura, J. L. (2012). The necessity of multiple test methods in conducting assessments: The role of the Rorschach and self-report. *Psychological Injury and Law, 5*(2), 97–106. https://doi.org/10.1007/s12207-012-9132-9

Mihura, J. L., Meyer, G. J., Dumitrascu, N., & Bombel, G. (2013). The validity of individual Rorschach variables: Systematic reviews and meta-analyses of the comprehensive system. *Psychological Bulletin, 139*(3), 548–605. https://doi.org/10.1037/a0029406

Millon, T. (2011). *Disorders of personality* (3rd ed.). John Wiley & Sons.

Morf, C. C., & Rhodewalt, F. (2001). Unraveling the paradoxes of narcissism: A dynamic self-regulatory processing model. *Psychological Inquiry, 12*(4), 177–196. https://doi.org/10.1207/S15327965PLI1204_1

Morf, C. C., Torchetti, L., & Schürch, E. (2011). Narcissism from the perspective of the dynamic self-regulatory processing model. In W. K. Campbell & J. D. Miller (Eds.), *The handbook of narcissism and narcissistic personality disorder: Theoretical approaches, empirical findings, and treatments* (pp. 56–70). John Wiley & Sons.

Pincus, A. L., & Lukowitsky, M. R. (2010). Pathological narcissism and narcissistic personality disorder. *Annual Review of Clinical Psychology, 6*, 421–446. https://doi.org/10.1146/annurev.clinpsy.121208.131215

Ronningstam, E. (2011). Narcissistic personality disorder in DSM V: In support of retaining a significant diagnosis. *Journal of Personality Disorders, 25*(2), 248–259. https://doi.org/10.1521/pedi.2011.25.2.248

Rorschach, H. (1921). *Psychodiagnostik* [Psychodiagnostics]. Bircher.

Ruggero, C. J., Kotov, R., Hopwood, C. J., First, M., Clark, L. A., Skodol, A. E., Mullins-Sweatt, S. N., Patrick, C. J., Bach, B., Cicero, D. C., Docherty, A., Simms, L. J., Bagby, R. M., Krueger, R. F., Callahan, J. L., Chmielewski, M., Conway, C. C., De Clercq, B., Dornbach-Bender, A., . . . Zimmermann, J. (2019). Integrating the Hierarchical Taxonomy of Psychopathology (HiTOP) into clinical practice. *Journal of Consulting and Clinical Psychology, 87*(12), 1069–1084. https://doi.org/10.1037/ccp0000452

Smith, J., Weinberger-Katzav, Y., & Fontan, P. (Eds.). (2022). *The Rorschach comprehensive system, revised supplementary scales handbook*. Rorschach Workshops.

Sommers-Flanagan, J. (2016). Clinical interview. In J. C. Norcross, G. R. VandenBos, D. K. Freedheim, & R. Krishnamurthy (Eds.), *APA handbook of clinical psychology: Applications and methods* (pp. 3–16). American Psychological Association.

Spring, B. (2007). Evidence-based practice in clinical psychology: What it is, why it matters; what you need to know. *Journal of Clinical Psychology, 63*(7), 611–631. https://doi.org/10.1002/jclp.20373

Stoyanov, D., Telles-Correia, D., & Cuthbert, B. N. (2019). The Research Domain Criteria (RDoC) and the historical roots of psychopathology: A viewpoint. *European Psychiatry, 57*, 58–60. https://doi.org/10.1016/j.eurpsy.2018.11.007

Van Laer, I. M. L., Vanhoyland, M., & De Saeger, H. (2020). Implementation of the Rorschach in an evidence-based setting: A Sisyphean task?! *Rorschachiana, 41*(2), 107–119. https://doi.org/10.1027/1192-5604/a000126

Weiner, I. B. & Kleiger, J. H. (Eds.). (2021). *Psychological assessment of disordered thinking and perception.* American Psychological Association.

Widiger, T. A. (2019). Considering the research: Commentary on "The trait–type dialectic: Construct validity, clinical utility, and the diagnostic process." *Personality Disorders: Theory, Research, and Treatment, 10*(3), 215–219. https://doi.org/10.1037/per0000322

Wilshire, C. E., Ward, T., & Clack, S. (2021). Symptom descriptions in psychopathology: How well are they working for us? *Clinical Psychological Science, 9*(3), 323–339. https://doi.org/10.1177/2167702620969215

Wilson, T. D., & Dunn, E. W. (2004). Self-knowledge: Its limits, value and potential for improvement. *Annual Review of Psychology, 55,* 493–518. https://doi.org/10.1146/annurev.psych.55.090902.141954

World Health Organization. (1994). *International classification of diseases* (10th ed.).

World Health Organization. (2019). *International classification of diseases* (11th ed.).

Yager, J., & McIntyre, J. S. (2014). DSM-5 Clinical and Public Health Committee: Challenges and considerations. *American Journal of Psychiatry, 171*(2), 142–144. https://doi.org/10.1176/appi.ajp.2013.13030347

Youngstrom, E. A., Choukas-Bradley, S., Calhoun, C. D., & Jensen-Doss, A. (2015). Clinical guide to the evidence-based assessment approach to diagnosis and treatment. *Cognitive and Behavioral Practice, 22*(1), 20–35. https://doi.org/10.1016/j.cbpra.2013.12.005

Zachar, P., & First, M. B. (2015). Transitioning to a dimensional model of personality disorder in DSM-5.1 and beyond. *Current Opinion in Psychiatry, 28*(1), 66–72. https://doi.org/10.1097/YCO.0000000000000115

Zeigler-Hill, V., Myers, E. M., & Clark, C. B. (2010). Narcissism and self-esteem reactivity: The role of negative achievement events. *Journal of Research in Personality, 44*(2), 285–292. https://doi.org/10.1016/j.jrp.2010.02.005

History
Received September 3, 2022
Revision received September 5, 2022
Accepted September 5, 2022
Published online October 21, 2022

Acknowledgments
This is an invited submission based on the author's Keynote address given at the International Society of the Rorschach and Projective Methods Centenary Congress in Geneva, Switzerland, July 11–15, 2022.

Conflict of Interest
The author reports no conflicts of interest related to this article.

ORCID
Robert F. Bornstein
https://orcid.org/0000-0001-6203-225X

Robert F. Bornstein
Derner School of Psychology
212 Blodgett Hall
Adelphi University
Garden City, NY 11530
USA
bornstein@adelphi.edu

Summary

To improve future versions of the diagnostic manuals we must expand the range of assessment methods that are used by clinicians to render psychiatric diagnoses. This article presents an evidence-based framework for integrating information derived from diagnostic interviews with data from the Rorschach Inkblot Method (RIM) to enhance diagnostic precision, improve treatment planning, and provide a novel paradigm for studying the dynamics of psychopathology in clinical and community settings. Use of multimethod assessment to inform diagnosis can help minimize diagnostic inaccuracies and biases that stem from the patient, from the diagnostician, and from the patient-diagnostician interaction. To do this effectively, it is important to have a clear understanding of the psychological processes that are engaged by interviews, and those that are engaged by the Rorschach. Using this information, the diagnostician can integrate interview and Rorschach data via three steps: 1) identify the underlying dynamics, expressed behaviors, and self-attributions associated with a particular disorder; 2) assess patient functioning in all three domains; and 3) interpret assessment results with attention to cross-method convergences and divergences. In addition to employing this three-step approach, implementing evidence-based multimethod diagnosis in clinical settings may require changes in the diagnostic systems. In future versions of the diagnostic manuals, each symptom should be explicitly identified according to the level of functioning that is captured by that symptom: underlying dynamics, self-attributions, or expressed behaviors. Evidence confirms that this process-focused framework can be employed to render trait-based diagnoses using the same logic, and same assessment strategies, as are used when diagnoses are rendered within the context of a categorical diagnostic system. As we move Rorschach's pioneering "research experiment" into its second century, it will be important to expand the range of settings in which RIM data are used; by doing this we can set the stage for continued interest in the Rorschach among clinicians, and among researchers as well.

Résumé

Pour améliorer les futures versions des manuels de diagnostic, nous devons élargir la gamme des méthodes d'évaluation utilisées par les cliniciens pour établir des diagnostics psychiatriques. Cet article présente un cadre fondé sur des données probantes pour l'intégration d'informations dérivées d'entretiens de diagnostic avec des données de la méthode Rorschach Inkblot (RIM) afin d'améliorer la précision du diagnostic, d'améliorer la planification du traitement et de fournir un nouveau paradigme pour étudier la dynamique de la psychopathologie en milieu clinique et communautaire. L'utilisation d'une évaluation multiméthode pour éclairer le diagnostic peut aider à minimiser les inexactitudes et les biais de diagnostic qui découlent du patient, du diagnosticien et de l'interaction patient-diagnosticien. Pour le faire efficacement, il est important d'avoir une compréhension claire des processus psychologiques qui sont engagés par les entretiens, et ceux qui sont engagés par le Rorschach. À l'aide de ces informations, le diagnosticien peut intégrer les données d'entretien et de Rorschach en trois étapes: 1) identifier la dynamique sous-jacente, les comportements exprimés et les auto-attributions associées à un trouble particulier; 2) évaluer le fonctionnement du patient dans les trois domaines; et 3) interpréter les résultats de l'évaluation en prêtant attention aux convergences et aux divergences entre les méthodes. En plus d'employer cette approche en trois étapes, la mise en œuvre d'un diagnostic multiméthode fondé sur des preuves dans les milieux cliniques peut nécessiter des changements dans les systèmes de diagnostic. Dans les futures versions des manuels de diagnostic, chaque symptôme devrait être explicitement identifié en fonction du niveau de fonctionnement qui est capturé par ce symptôme: dynamique sous-jacente, auto-attributions ou comportements exprimés. Les preuves confirment que ce cadre axé sur les processus peut être utilisé pour rendre des diagnostics basés sur les traits en utilisant la même logique et les mêmes stratégies d'évaluation que celles utilisées lorsque les diagnostics sont rendus dans le contexte d'un système de diagnostic catégoriel. Alors que nous avançons « l'expérience de recherche » pionnière de Rorschach dans son deuxième siècle, il sera important d'élargir la gamme de paramètres dans lesquels les données RIM sont utilisées; ce faisant, nous pouvons ouvrir la voie à un intérêt continu pour le Rorschach parmi les cliniciens, ainsi que parmi les chercheurs.

Resumen

Para mejorar las versiones futuras de los manuales de diagnóstico, debemos ampliar la gama de métodos de evaluación que utilizan los médicos para realizar diagnósticos psiquiátricos. Este artículo presenta un marco basado en evidencia para integrar información derivada de entrevistas diagnósticas con datos del método de manchas de tinta de Rorschach (RIM) para mejorar la precisión diagnóstica, mejorar la planificación del tratamiento y proporcionar un paradigma novedoso para estudiar la dinámica de la psicopatología en entornos clínicos y comunitarios. El uso de la evaluación multimétodo para informar el diagnóstico puede ayudar a minimizar las inexactitudes y los sesgos de diagnóstico que se derivan del paciente, del diagnosticador y de la interacción paciente-diagnosticador. Para hacer esto de manera efectiva, es importante tener una comprensión clara de los procesos psicológicos que involucran las entrevistas y los que involucra el Rorschach. Usando esta información, el diagnosticador puede integrar la entrevista y los datos de Rorschach a través de tres pasos: 1) identificar la dinámica subyacente, los comportamientos expresados y las autoatribuciones asociadas con un trastorno en particular; 2) evaluar el funcionamiento del paciente en los tres dominios; y 3) interpretar los resultados de la evaluación con atención a las convergencias y divergencias entre métodos. Además de emplear este enfoque de tres pasos, la implementación de diagnósticos multimétodo basados en evidencia en entornos clínicos puede requerir cambios en los sistemas de diagnóstico. En versiones futuras de los manuales de diagnóstico, cada síntoma debe identificarse explícitamente de acuerdo con el nivel de funcionamiento que capta ese síntoma: dinámica subyacente, autoatribuciones o comportamientos expresados. La evidencia confirma que este marco centrado en el proceso se puede emplear para generar diagnósticos basados en rasgos usando la misma lógica y las mismas estrategias de evaluación que se usan cuando los diagnósticos se presentan dentro del contexto de un sistema de diagnóstico categórico. A medida que avanzamos en el "experimento de investigación" pionero de Rorschach hacia su segundo siglo, será importante ampliar la gama de entornos en los que se utilizan los datos RIM; Al hacer esto, podemos preparar el escenario para un interés continuo en el Rorschach entre los médicos y también entre los investigadores.

要約

診断マニュアルをより良いものにするためには、臨床医が精神科診断に用いる評価方法の幅を広げることが必要である。本稿では、診断的な面接から得られた情報とロールシャッハ・インクブロット法（RIM）のデータを統合することで、診断の精度を高め、治療計画を改善し、臨床および地域社会における精神病理のダイナミクスを研究するための新しいパラダイムを提供するためのエビデンスに基づく枠組みを提示する。多面的評価を診断に活用することで、患者、診断者、患者-診断者間の相互作用に起因する診断の不正確さや偏りを最小限に抑えることができる。これを効果的に行うには、面接が関与する心理過程とロールシャッハが関与する心理過程を明確に理解することが重要である。この情報をもとに、診断者は3つのステップを経て、インタビューとロールシャッハのデータを統合することができる。その3つのステップとは、次の

通りである。1）根底にある力動、表出行動、自己帰属のような特定の疾患に関連することを特定する、2）3つの領域すべてにおいて患者の機能を評価する、3）方法間の収束と拡散に注意しながら評価結果を解釈する。この3ステップのアプローチを採用することに加え、臨床の場でエビデンスに基づいた多方面からの診断を実施するには、診断システムの変更が必要かもしれない。将来的にこの診断マニュアルでは、各症状はその症状によって捉えられる機能のレベル（根底にある力動、自己帰属、表出行動）に従って明示的に同定されるべきであろう。このプロセス重視の枠組みは、カテゴリー診断システムの文脈の中で診断がなされた時と同じ論理と同じ評価戦略を用いて、特性ベースの診断を下すために用いることができるというエビデンスによって確認されている。ロールシャッハの「研究実験」が世に出て2世紀目を迎えた今、RIMデータの利用範囲を広げることが重要である。そうすることで、臨床家だけでなく研究者の間でもロールシャッハへの関心が高まり続けるだろう。

Special Issue: New Insights From Other Psychological Disciplines for
Rorschach Users
Original Article

The Active Bayesian Brain and the Rorschach Task

Gregory J. Meyer[1] and Karl J. Friston[2]

[1]Department of Psychology, University of Toledo, OH, USA
[2]The Wellcome Centre for Human Neuroimaging, UCL Queen Square Institute of Neurology,
University College London, UK

Abstract: The Rorschach offers a unique and interesting paradigm from the perspective of the (Bayesian) brain. This contribution to the cross-disciplinary special issue considers the Rorschach from the perspective of perceptual inference in the brain and how it might inform subject-specific differences in perceptual synthesis. Before doing so, we provide a broad overview of active inference in its various manifestations. In brief, active inference supposes that our perceptions are the best hypothesis to explain sensory impressions. On a Bayesian account, the requisite belief updating rests sensitively upon the precision or confidence ascribed to sensory input, relative to prior beliefs about the causes of sensations. This focus – on the balance between sensory and prior precision – has been a useful construct in both cognitive science (e.g., as a formal explanation for attention) and neuropsychology (e.g., as a formal explanation for aberrant or false inference in hallucinations). In this setting, false inference is generally understood as abnormally high precision afforded to high-level hypotheses or explanations for visual input, which may compensate for a failure to attenuate sensory precision. On this view, the Rorschach offers an interesting paradigm because the amount of precise information about the causes of visual input is deliberately minimized – and rendered ambiguous – thereby placing greater emphasis on prior beliefs entertained by the respondent. We close by exploring this issue and several other areas of intersection between Rorschach responding and active inference.

Keywords: active inference, Rorschach assessment, Bayesian probability, visual perception

This essay begins broadly, providing readers with the backdrop for active inference, focusing on how active inference is founded on Bayesian probabilities and functions as a formal model for how human minds work. This part of the exposition draws on work by Friston (2009, 2013), Friston et al. (2012), and particularly Parr et al. (2022). Interested readers will find sources such as Clark (2013, 2016), Hohwy (2016), Barrett (2017), Otten et al. (2017), and Wiese and Metzinger (2017) to be useful entrées to the key ideas. With this review as foundation, we address our ultimate aim, which is to consider how the Bayesian brain may evince an understanding of the processes engaged when a person sits with an assessor to participate in the inkblot task developed by Hermann Rorschach.

Rorschachiana (2022), 43(2), 128–150
https://doi.org/10.1027/1192-5604/a000158

However, before getting to those topics, we first briefly review Bayesian probabilities. Thomas Bayes (~1701–1761) was a British minister and statistician who developed a relatively simple equation to convert one's current belief about an outcome or event (E; called the prior probability) into a revised and updated belief (called the posterior probability) after encountering some new piece of information, which can be considered a sensory sign or signal (S). The result (i.e., the posterior probability) is a conditional probability because it depends on (i.e., is conditioned on) the new piece of information (i.e., it is E given S, or in symbols E | S). Although most resources present the calculations for Bayes theorem using proportions, Bayes did not and the math is simpler to understand using frequencies (e.g., Gigerenzer & Hoffrage, 1995). To compute the updated conditional probability, one needs to know how often the outcome or event occurs in the presence of the signal (E&S) and how often the signal shows up naturally (S). With those two pieces of information, the posterior probability is simply E&S / S. For instance, say it rains (E) on cloudy days (S) 3 times per month (i.e., E&S = 3) and it is cloudy 9 days per month (i.e., S = 9). On any given day, one's confidence it will rain that day (i.e., prior probability) is roughly 10% (i.e., 3 / ~30). However, if it is cloudy that day, one's confidence it will rain (the posterior probability, E | S) is 33% (i.e., 3 / 9).

The Bayesian Brain

The Broad View

All living organisms face the same challenge: to maintain separateness or boundedness from their surrounding environment. Maintaining separateness is essential to permit efforts toward sustenance and reproduction, as without separateness organisms would dissolve into their surroundings by the forces of entropy (i.e., natural disorder, disorganization, dissipation, and death), per the second law of thermodynamics. Further, all organisms evolved to persist in, or exploit, a relatively narrow band of preferred physiological or characteristic states out of all those available, so that all organisms must also avoid those states that are poorly suited to their existential needs (e.g., fish need to live in water, but also need to avoid waters beyond their preferred temperature range and salinity).

According to the model on offer, organisms fulfil their particular aims by actively minimizing the likelihood of encountering environmental circumstances that generate unexpected sensory states, which are conceptualized as "surprising" sensory observations. Surprise in this context has a technical meaning (in information theory it is called self information), in that it indexes the extent to which the source of its current sensory input differs from expected or preferred sensory inputs that are conducive to the persistence of the organism. Because it is generally impossible for an organism to know the true causes of its sensations, minimizing surprise itself is an intractable problem; so instead, organisms minimize an approximation to it called free energy. Free energy, like surprise, is an index of entropic mismatch between an organism's preferred states and its current sensory samples of the environment. Crucially, free energy is determined just by the organism's expected or preferred states and their sensory experience of the environment at the moment, which, of course, is just a proxy for the actual environmental causes of that sensation.

Separateness and boundedness are not just requirements of organisms, but also are required for any organized, adaptive system. Within an organism there may be many organized systems (e.g., a brain encased within a skull, a vascular system throughout the body). For each, there is a boundary individuating it from its surroundings. What is on the other side of that boundary is hidden from that within the boundary (e.g., the external environment is inaccessible for a brain in a skull). Statistically, the boundary functions as what is known as a Markov blanket, which mediates between outer states and inner states; namely, states that are external to the system and those that are internal to it. From the perspective of active inference, the internal system has only two options for inferring what is outside of the system, both of which are mediated via the blanket; the blanket can mediate action from within to without (via active states such as muscles and autonomic reflexes) and it can sample the environment (via sensory states such as sensory epithelia and receptors) from without to within. However, the internal states of the system cannot directly influence the outer states and vice versa; inner influences outer only through active states (e.g., actions) and outer influences inner only through sensory states (e.g., observations). Together, the active and sensory states constitute blanket states.

The term blanket comes from the idea of enclosing or enveloping. In human terms, a Markov blanket would be one's outer surface, which is largely skin, although the term skin is generally not used for the inner parts of the mouth, nose, or ears. To know what resides outside oneself, the action options include to look, listen, sniff, taste, touch, move (ambulate), or think. The options to sense outside the body are mainly through the eyes, ears, nose, mouth, and skin, using sensory mechanisms that have an adaptively limited range of functions to detect what is truly external to the self (e.g., people cannot smell like dogs, hear like bats, or use magnetism like birds).

In any adaptive system capable of persisting, active states and sensory states have a reciprocal or symmetrical relationship with each other, in that active states influence outer states and outer states respond by providing updated sensory states for the organism. This permits the organism (the inner state) to update conditional Bayesian probabilities to infer its external states and thus make probabilistic inferences about the causes of its sensations (e.g., a finger stroke on an object generates a sensation of roughness, increasing the probability of it being a certain type of hidden cause and lowering the probability of it being others). Those internal inferences update Bayesian prior probabilities or initial expectations that then form the baseline for what to expect from the environment or niche as the organism acts to sample it further. Those inferences thus serve to foster what can be understood as a model or representation of the external environment, reducing its uncertainty and implicitly, actively reducing the unpredictability of the external states of affairs in the niche.

In short, this reduction helps minimize free energy, which is an index of unexpected environmental surprises that generally counter adaptive persistence. For instance, a fish that swims left yet senses a large shadow moving similarly overhead may associate that sensation with an increased likelihood (i.e., probability) of danger, which should increase in certainty further if it then swims away and the shadow follows. Thus, although they vary tremendously in their complexity, adaptive systems form a type of "understanding" or recognition of their environment through their bounded exchange with that environment. From an active inference perspective, this type of recognition unfolds via a process of Bayesian belief updating, under a generative model.

Generative models do more than track linked patterns of active and sensory states. They serve both as a probabilistic base of inference (i.e., Bayesian prior probability) and as a mechanism to advance the needs of the inner state in order for the organism to persist over time. Further, the generative model encompasses the intrinsic needs of the organism; in the sense that those intrinsically preferred, adaptive states form a core base set of prior probabilities for that organism. These core prior probabilities guide the organism to find itself in just that niche, such that it literally perceives itself to be in – and acts to get in – environmental states that are conducive to its survival. Doing so reduces the mismatch between the organism's predictions generated by its internal model and its sensations (i.e., it minimizes free energy).

A generative model can be quite simple, or it can be organized into greater degrees of complexity, with multiple factors, modules, modalities, and domains; each serving distinct subsystems for the organism (e.g., temperature regulation vs. response to threat). In addition, increasingly complex generative models are hierarchically organized to permit organisms to make inferences across different timescales and to subserve distinct preferences or expected states. Systems with the capacity to model alternative courses of action and their predicted consequences, and to correspondingly be able to engage their environments with agency, likely form the foundation for all sentient organisms, including people.

These systems need not just minimize free energy in the moment (*variational* free energy), but also minimize the free energy associated with different possible courses of action in the future (*expected* free energy). The distinction here is between something like determining if you should put another layer of clothing on now to counter an emerging chill (minimize variational free energy) and deciding if it is worth the effort to carry an umbrella to counter a potential chill from rain later (minimizing expected free energy).

All life forms – and any adaptive system that actively samples its sensory states to minimize variational free energy – entails a generative model. In this formulation a generative model is simply a probabilistic representation that can guide some form of action, including something as simple as secreting a chemical. Such systems can retain their boundaries, regulate their internal states, and persist in an environment suited to their particular life needs. However, the distinction between variational and expected free energy offers a "bright line" between simpler life forms, which exist solely in the present (even if they have future-oriented adaptations, such as trees that drop their leaves annually), and more complex life forms that can explicitly plan and select among possible alternative futures. The latter permits at least some level of deliberation, agency, and sentience.

The Focused View

Active inference in sentient organisms operates using hierarchical Bayesian predictive coding, where specialized neuronal paths send predictions of what to expect from higher cortical levels via representation unit neurons to the lower levels, ultimately reaching the sensory epithelia. In this hierarchical or deep architecture, each level conveys predictions to the next level down. Return signals from the sense receptors then traverse each layer of the hierarchy, but do so using error unit neurons. These neurons convey prediction errors or "surprising" information that is not explained by the downward flowing predictions. These prediction errors inform top–down cells at their level and at the level directly above. (This process of returning residuals [i.e., predicted experience – encountered experience = prediction error] rather than already known information is efficient metabolically and somewhat analogous to lossless file compression techniques, which discard predictable information [e.g., .png or .zip file formats]). Importantly, predictions or prior beliefs (i.e., Bayesian prior probabilities) are themselves probability distributions, not point estimates, meaning for every representation an organism has – of the hidden environmental causes of their sensations – there is an expectation (i.e., mean) and an associated degree of confidence or precision (i.e., variance) that determines the degree of certainty with which they are held. High confidence produces a narrow, peaked distribution, while low confidence produces a broad and flat distribution. Similarly, sensory inputs, and the degree of prediction error they return to trigger a revision of predictions (i.e., Bayesian posterior probabilities) or affirm a match with prior predictions, also are probabilistic, with their magnitude (mean) and precision (variance) determined by the quality and reliability of the sensory signal. In short, each level in the hierarchy encodes the uncertainty or precision associated with its current (Bayesian) beliefs that affects both the top–down predictions and the bottom–up errors. This precision is thought to be mediated by the frequency and intensity of the synaptic signals at each juncture. More specifically, precision may be encoded by the sensitivity of prediction error units to their inputs; such that a high degree of precision at one level of the hierarchy means that the prediction errors have a greater influence on belief updating at superior levels. Physiologically, this corresponds to synaptic gain, while psychologically, it can be regarded as an implementation of attentional gain – or its attenuation.

Each level of this hierarchical structure seeks to reconcile or cancel or resolve prediction errors to reduce uncertainty and optimize its representation of external states. Note that minimizing prediction errors is just the same as minimizing free energy or surprise as noted in our treatment of adaptive exchange with the environment above. Importantly, agents can amplify certain prediction errors by focusing attention on the signals provided, or they can inhibit that input to attenuate messages. For instance, sensory attenuation is required for an agent to take any action, because any effort to move would be countered otherwise by error signals conveying that in fact that movement is not taking place. The constant interplay of the predictions and prediction errors, up and down the neural hierarchy, leaves considerable room for problems to develop in the sensorium, such that prior beliefs may be inappropriately amplified or attenuated (higher or lower prior certainty) or held too tentatively or confidently (wide or narrow prior precision or variance). The same is true with respect to sensory input, which can be inappropriately strong or weak (higher or lower sensory signal) or dismissed or amplified (wide or narrow distribution). For instance, one could feel more or less hungry than is true physiologically (incorrectly high or low signals) and one could be uncertain or very confident about that level of hunger (incorrectly wide or narrow signals).

At the same time, it is quite adaptive, in the right context, to give excess weight to one level of hierarchal processing or another. Highly weighted sensory signals can quickly update one's (Bayesian or subpersonal) beliefs about the environment, which can be helpful when in novel or dangerous surroundings, changing or chaotic circumstances, or if the signal is particularly strong and precise. Highly weighted prior predictions are stubbornly resistant to change and influence, which can be helpful when operating under stable and familiar conditions or when the environmental signals are vague, contradictory, or confusing.

Thus, the active inference model, in its broadest form, posits that all creatures seek to find and make niches over momentary and lifelong time frames that minimize prediction error about the hidden external causes of sensation, as that error is a manifestation of the deleterious and dissipative forces of entropy (i.e., unpredictability is a manifestation of disorder or randomness in the life trajectory of the organism). They do so by constantly predicting what the agent should experience and sense and constantly affirming or updating those predictions based on the error notifications from the senses.

Active inference itself is the process of resolving discrepancies between one's model of experience (i.e., prior predictions) and the sensations generated by actual but hidden environmental signals. One can do this either by taking some action (e.g., allocate attention, step back, shift gaze, smell more deeply, turn an ear, touch again) to resample sensory information to confirm the prediction or by letting error signals override and correct the generative model of prediction. Changing one's mind to accommodate updated beliefs is *perception*. Modifying the environment sensed or sampled is *action*. Active inference thus leads either to *affirmation* of the prediction via action bringing affirming sensory samples with minimal prediction error or to *correction* to foster a refined prediction that resolves prediction errors via perception – and that is now accompanied by new recognition. Both paths serve the aim of minimizing the discrepancy between one's model of the environment and the environment itself (i.e., minimize free energy). It is easy to find illustrations of these ideas through common expressions that often emerge in conversation using terminology for embodied cognition. For instance, a listener may exclaim, "Oh, I see!" as a manifestation of perception (i.e., arriving at a new corrected understanding or view) or a speaker may offer guidance for action by saying, "No, look at it this way; ..." or "Consider it from this perspective; ..." directing the listener to mentally move to a different position to see their point.

The Conventional View

Although there is much more that could be said about active inference and the Bayesian brain, this overview sketches out its main features. The view that the brain is fundamentally a prediction machine dates back to Helmholtz in the 1860s. However, it is worth highlighting how this model of minds, brains, and nervous systems is in contrast to the alternative view that has been conventional for decades. That view is of sensory cells taking in specific features of the environment and using the neural hierarchy to build at higher cortical levels an increasingly complex and accurate understanding of what is being perceived (e.g.,

Aggelopoulos, 2015). Rather than viewing perception as a one-way process of passively taking in sensory information and then trying to figure it out, the actively inferring Bayesian brain begins with a generative model that uses an active, constructive process going from the inside out. As such, sensations of and from the environment – which are shaped, shifted, and refined by the agent's actions – serve to affirm or modify the organism's model of the hidden causes behind those sensations. Complex agents infer the source of their experiential sensations, with experiential sensation encompassing the world of objects and actions outside oneself and the similarly remote or hidden world of processes, impulses, affects, and needs inside one's own body.

Empirical Grounding and Applications of the Model

The active inference model encompasses many facets. However, they are all grounded in rigorously defined mathematical formalisms that are tightly linked to biologically plausible mechanisms of action in the context of evolutionary developments for all living organisms, sentient or not. The paradigm has been remarkably heuristic (Clark, 2016; Parr et al., 2022), providing guidelines for more advanced robotics and artificial intelligence, as well as explaining brain localization and functions and their proclivity for using specific neurotransmitters. Within psychological concerns more specifically, these models are being used to conceptualize topics as diverse as psychedelic experiences (Carhart-Harris, 2018), hypnosis (Martin & Pacherie, 2019), interoception (e.g., Seth, 2013), attention (e.g., Parr & Friston, 2017), trauma (e.g., Linson et al., 2020), schizophrenia (e.g., Friston et al., 2016), hallucinations (e.g., Benrimoh et al., 2018), delusions (e.g., Adams et al., 2014), autism (e.g., Palmer et al., 2017), movement disorders (e.g., Brown et al., 2013), Freud's unfinished *Project for a Scientific Psychology* (Carhart-Harris & Friston, 2010), and consciousness itself (Solms & Friston, 2018), to name a few.

Links to Engaging With the Rorschach Task

With this as backdrop, we turn to consider several ways in which active inference can be applied to Rorschach's inkblot task. In particular, we attempt to make links with some of Rorschach's own views of what the task was, how it worked, and, in consequence, what it provided. For those views, we rely heavily on the excellent and substantially clearer new English translation of his work by Keddy, Signer, Erdberg, and Schneider-Stocking (Rorschach, 1921/2021).

Key Features of the Task

As readers of this journal know, the Rorschach is a performance task that relies on visual–spatial and lexical–conceptual problem solving, using the standard set of 10 vertically symmetrical inkblot designs set on white cardstock. Five are shades of gray, two are shades of gray with prominent bold red areas, and three are fully chromatic with elements ranging from pleasing pastels to brightly saturated colors. For administration, the assessor hands respondents each card in order, while asking the question, "What might this be?" Respondents typically reply with two or three responses per card and their replies represent their personal solutions to deciphering the problem at hand. Subsequently, the assessor goes back through the cards and clarifies where objects reside and what inkblot features contributed to that perception. Finally, most assessors then classify each response across multiple dimensions (e.g., use of color, envisioning human activity, coherence of thought processes), and aggregate the codes across all responses to form summary scores capable of contrasting the respondent to what most people see, say, and do when completing the task.

Although likely less well known to many readers, the inkblots are not random designs, despite Rorschach referring to them in the subtitle to his text as "accidental forms." To the contrary, Rorschach used his artistic training to carefully create, pilot-test, and artistically refine each card over time to ensure they would not simply look like inkblots (Rorschach, 1921/2021; Searls, 2017). In fact, the Rorschach Archives contain multiple iterations of each of the 10 cards that are clearly recognizable but differ from the final version in their accentuation of features and their overall composition. Of this iterative process, Rorschach (1921/2021, p. 4) said, "The picture series used in the test gradually developed on the basis of empirical observation."

He appears to have had two intertwined aims when developing them, both based on the suggestive "critical bits" (Exner, 1996) that encompass the prominent inkblot areas and shapes and also their color, shading, irregular interior and exterior contours, and subtly imbalanced symmetrical features. First, within the designed composition of each card, he embedded at least one reasonably recognizable object or part of an object to form the commonly reported conventional percepts (e.g., the human-like figures on Card III and the animal-like figures on Card VIII). Second, he embedded a textured array of other features that contradict or complicate the more recognizable elements (e.g., a part looks pretty clearly like a person's head, but what would be its torso looks more like the head of a horned creature).

These opposing qualities produce evocative but incomplete or imperfect perceptual likenesses that (deliberately and artfully) stimulate uncertainty, ambiguity, and imprecision among the competing visual impressions that may underwrite potential responses. They also provide a task with considerable embedded structure, as well as a wide array of alternative features that idiographically hook perception and contribute to personally unique perceptions. The embedded structure provides a mechanism for assessing conventionality in the locations selected for percepts (i.e., the focus of one's attention; Berry & Meyer, 2019) and the quality of the fit of objects to those locations (i.e., perceptual accuracy as coded by Form Quality). The idiographic diversity provides personally salient, experience-near imagery that can richly illustrate the respondent's psychological processing. Interestingly, even in very large samples, unique objects seen by just a single person account for about 70% of all the distinct objects reported (Meyer et al., 2011). For instance, Villemor-Amaral and her colleagues (2007) identified a total of 6,459 response objects in a sample of 600 nonpatients. The most common object was identified by 375 people and just 30 objects were seen by 50 or more people; however, 4,538 objects were identified by just one person.

The task of dealing with imprecision in the provocative and deliberately contradictory stimuli, as well as uncertainty regarding the adequacy of one's responses, occurs in an interpersonal context while the respondent interacts with a relative stranger (sitting adjacent) who is observing and transcribing the exchange. These features make the task moderately stressful, and more physiologically stressful than assessment by other methods, such as self-report (e.g., Momenian-Schneider et al., 2009; Newmark et al., 1974, 1975).

For the respondent, solving the problem of what the inkblot might be invokes a series of perceptual and problem-solving (belief updating) processes. These include scanning the stimuli, selecting locations for potential response objects, comparing potential inkblot images to objects in memory, evaluating possible percepts relative to their inconsistencies or contradictions, reformulating response options, filtering out those judged less optimal, and articulating a final solution to the assessor (Exner, 2003). The respondent's visual-mnemonic matching of objects in the card to recalled images, conceptual processing of the stimuli, and verbal and nonverbal communication engage all brain regions, encompassing bilateral activity in the frontal, temporal, parietal, occipital, and limbic lobes (e.g., Asari et al., 2008, 2010a, 2010b; Giromini et al., 2017).

Psychological Processes Engaged

The available neurophysiological data indicate that completing the task engages both the dorsal and ventral attentional systems (Giromini et al., 2017). The dorsal system is important for directing conceptually guided top-down attentional search processes (i.e., predictions of what it might be) and the ventral system is important for recognizing and reorienting to surprising or unexpected bottom–up input (e.g., misfits with prediction, alternative possibilities). These two attentional systems are negatively correlated with the default mode network (e.g., Zhou et al., 2018), which in humans is implicated in self-referential processing, including the intro-spective attribution of self-reported characteristics (e.g., Davey et al., 2016).

These data on Rorschach responding fit nicely with an active Bayesian brain, as the respondent is iteratively refining the fit of conceptual priors (beliefs about what it might be, carried by the dorsal attention system) to environmental (visual) stim-uli with an uncertain or ambiguous cause. Given their intentionally contradictory features, the Rorschach images consistently provide the viewer with irreducible error signals that the prediction is not quite right and is evincing ill-fitting incon-gruities (ventral attention system). Respondents reduce this prediction error to modify the initial prediction about what is "out there" in the environment (i.e., by changing one's mind about the percept) or by taking actions to sample the envi-ronment (e.g., shift gaze, modify location boundaries) and more precisely affirm the prediction (i.e., by gathering better evidence). This results in an iterative cal-ibration process that ultimately provides the respondent's error-corrected, person-alized perceptual equilibrium (i.e., beliefs) about the hidden features of the environment. Of course, here the inkblots are serving as analogs to the parallel processes occurring when encountering the many ambiguities of daily life (Clark, 2016).

In other words, the Rorschach task presents a carefully designed and special problem for perceptual inference, in that there is no single perceptual explanation that fully accounts for the visual information at hand. This provides an unprece-dented tool to explore the landscape of a subject's prior beliefs about the causes of their sensations. In one sense, Rorschach's task is the ultimate tool for disclos-ing prior beliefs. It is reminiscent of how psychophysics reveals prior beliefs through the use of illusions: Illusory stimuli (e.g., ambiguous figures or stimuli that induce bistable perception) are carefully constructed to induce ambiguity, obliging the perceiver to explore and alternate between perceptual hypotheses that reveal the kind of hypotheses people use in everyday perceptual synthesis.

This ambiguity is not an accidental feature of Rorschach's task. He designed it to engage just this form of active inference to allow an assessor to see the mean-ing-making process in action. Rorschach (1921/2021) viewed the task as one of "perception and apperception" (p. 36), not imagination or gaining access to uncon-scious processes per se. He considered *perception* to be the outcome of an associa-tive process between sensation and one's memory of former sensations, paralleling how that term is used in active inference. *Apperception* was the process of linking sensory perceptions with their prior connections in order to understand current sensations based on past experience. This can be viewed as the process of getting to perception, which is active inference, or the process of balancing predictions and errors to "know" what is experienced. However, Rorschach (1921/2021) saw one big difference between those processes in everyday life and those processes when examining his inkblots; in essence, the inkblots slowed perception to render it visible:

> If perception [is] an associative *integration of present engrams* [memory traces] *with recent complexes of sensations*, then *the interpretation of accidental* [indeterminate] *forms can be called a perception in which the effort of integration of the sensations and the memory trace is so great that it is perceived as an effort of integration.* This intrapsychic perception of incomplete equality [i.e., discrepancy] between the complexes of sensation and the engram gives the perception the character of an interpretation. ... Most respondents with either schizophrenia, epilepsy, manic-depressive illness, or organic disorders... are not aware of the effort of integration. Even many normal respondents are not aware of it. These respondents do not interpret the pictures, they name them. They may even be astonished if other respondents see something different in them. In these cases, this is not an interpretation but rather a perception in the strict sense of the word. They are as unaware of the associative effort of integration as a normal person is when recognizing a familiar face or perceiving a tree. Therefore, there must be a kind of threshold beyond which perception (the integration without awareness of the effort of it) becomes interpretation (perception with awareness of the effort of integration). ... In summary, we may conclude that *the differences between perception and interpretation are based on individual and gradational factors, not on general, principal ones; thus, interpretation may be a special case of perception.* There is, therefore, no doubt that the form interpretation experiment [i.e., the inkblot task] can be called an investigation into perception. (pp. 36–37, italics in the original)

Thus, Rorschach recognized that the task, while one of perception, also helped show the iterative cycle of prediction, error correction, active search, revised prediction, further error correction, further action, and so on. Of course, this view is quite compatible with the iterative processes undertaken by the Bayesian brain.

Rorschach (1921/2021) provides further elaboration of his views on what the task does and does not provide later in the text, when discussing interpretation. He considered the extent to which respondents mentally enlivened their perceptions with human activity and the extent to which they recognized and incorporated the bright, vibrant coloration of the cards as key dimensions that differentiated individuals. However, he was clear that there was not a direct correspondence between the nature of one's perceptions and behavior in everyday life. Thus, after quantifying these two dimensions, Rorschach concluded that the assessor would "know a lot about the respondent" (p. 106). He further clarified that what the task revealed was the sensory–perceptual structures of the individual that registers their day-to-day experiences; revealing their lived experience but not the way they live their life:

> We do not know what this respondent experiences, but, rather, *how this respondent experiences*. We know a large part of the characteristics and dispositions with which the respondent goes through life, be they of an associative or affective nature or a mixture of the two. We do not know their experiences, but we do know the *experience apparatus* [also psychical apparatus] with which they receive experiences from the inside and from the outside, and to which the respondents initially subject their experiences to processing. (p. 106, italics in the original)

> The experience apparatus with which the individual experiences is a much broader, more extensive structure than the apparatus with which the individual lives. To experience, a person has a number of registers but only uses a few for the actions of life – often so few that it ends in stereotypy. The experience type [balance of movement to color] reveals how broad the apparatus is with which the respondent could live. It cannot reveal, however, actually – except under very favorable circumstances – what parts of the apparatus the respondent activates for active living. (p. 108)

Envisioning Human Action

Another domain in which the actively inferring Bayesian brain manifests in Rorschach responding is with respect to envisioning human activity. The mirror neuron system is activated when a person engages in a particular course of action and similarly activated when observing another person engaging in that particular course of action. It is viewed as the neuronal representation of understanding what others are doing (proprioceptive and exteroceptive) and why (goals and intentions) when we observe their behavior and actions in a particular context (e.g., Friston et al., 2011; Kilner et al., 2007). In essence, we use our experience of a movement or activity in context to understand another's movement or activity in that context, and this is done through active inference, mentally anticipating (predicting) the act and modifying the mental prediction based on mismatches (errors) between the observed and internally enacted action. On this basis, one could anticipate how seeing human activity in inkblot imagery would similarly activate the mirror neurons.

Indeed, Rorschach (1921/2021) anticipated as much when describing the human Movement code, *M*. "Movement responses (M) are those interpretations which are determined by *form perception plus kinesthetic factors*. The respondent imagines the object interpreted to be in motion" (p. 45, italics in the original). Thus, Rorschach was identifying an empathic, enactive internal response to the action perceived. Subsequent neurophysiological research using multiple methods (electroencephalography [EEG], transcranial magnetic stimulation [TMS], magnetic resonance imaging [MRI]) has affirmed these views, with clear evidentiary support that the mirror neuron system is activated when respondents produce responses coded *M*, but not when simply seeing static human figures or animals in action (see, e.g., Giromini et al., 2019).

Introversiveness and Motility: An Open Question

Rorschach was fascinated with movement, including its artistic depiction, its consequences for mental life, its manifestations in culture and cults, and, of course, in responses to his inkblots (Akavia, 2013). For the latter, he used his considerable skills depicting action in drawings and paintings to provide movement-suggestive stimuli in the inkblots in order to understand the type of person who responded to it. Rorschach (1921/2021) believed *M* responses required a degree of delay and reflection to formulate, reflecting a style of processing that was ideational and introversive (i.e., "capable of introversion"; p. 97). In contrast to the zeitgeist at the time (Akavia), he also believed there was an inverse relationship between physical movement and perceiving human movement in the inkblots:

> *The measure of the manifest motility in a respondent is not the measure of the kinesthesias* [responses with M] *influencing the respondent during the perception process. On the contrary, the kinesthetic individual is motorically stable; the lively person is poor in kinesthesias.* (p. 45, italics in the original)

And further, "Introversion ... is increased by an active shutting down of the factors that inhibit it and decreased by restarting the function of adaptation" (p. 97).

Indeed, among patients with schizophrenia, Rorschach (1921/2021) concluded that those with catatonia produced the highest number of responses coded *M* (Table 2, p. 42). Rorschach had extensive experience with patients who had schizophrenia and he wrote a lengthy unpublished case study of Theodor Niehans, a patient he assessed and treated at the Münsingen asylum, with a well-documented 20-year history at the asylum (Akavia, 2013). Over the years, Niehans went from profound paranoia to profound catatonia and back again. Akavia notes, "Rorschach ultimately conceptualized the catatonic form of schizophrenia, ostensibly a state of extreme stasis, as manifesting an intense internal dynamism of 'fettered movement'" (p. 6), which Niehans himself characterized as a period of "compulsive thought" (p. 121). In the case study, Rorschach contrasted paranoia and catatonia, saying, "the catatonic renounced the outside world and abandoned himself to introversion, while the paranoid resisted introversion by desperately cleaving to the outside world" (p. 106). Akavia concluded: "Rorschach... saw catatonia and its concomitant physical immobility as a mode of utmost mental excitability, whereby – at least in the case of Niehans – schizophrenic psychological activity found its consummate inward form, giving rise to an active, ongoing development of florid delusions" (p. 123).

Interestingly, Brown et al. (2013) used active inference to model the consequences of a compromised ability in the typical requirement to attenuate sensory signals during self-generated movement. This attenuation is required to initiate action and it is commonly compromised in patients with schizophrenia. Failing to attenuate those sensory signals leaves sensory signals stronger and more precise than one's predictions of movement; as such, sensory prediction errors predominate over top–down projections. Under these conditions, they observed profound impairment of movement, reminiscent of the psychomotor symptoms of catatonia. Although their modeling did not encompass ideational activity, it is a fascinating open question about whether these conditions would lead to an increased number of ideationally active human movement responses on the inkblot task, as Rorschach's observations suggest.

Rorschach's (1921/2021) notion that inkblots "slowed perception to render it visible" is exactly congruent with the definitive role of precision or uncertainty coding in the covert action associated with sensory attention and attenuation. This follows because the precision determines the rate of belief updating. In other words, assigning a greater weight to certain prediction errors means they have a greater influence on neural populations encoding expectations and subsequent predictions higher in the hierarchy. Precluding a precise, high-level prior explanation for sensory input will therefore preclude precise prediction errors higher in the visual (or more generally perceptual) hierarchies – and thereby attenuate the rate of belief updating or assimilation of prediction errors from lower levels. This corresponds exactly with the notion of slowing perceptual synthesis so that its architecture and fundaments can be disclosed through responses reported to the assessor.

Perceptual Distortions

Finally, we consider perceptual distortions, which from a Bayesian brain perspective may emerge from either end of the neural hierarchy, such that hallucinations and perceptual distortions may occur when sensory signals fail to be attenuated or perceptual priors are underweighted (e.g., Adams et al., 2013) or, more typically, when prior beliefs are overweighted and corrective sensory input is underweighted during percept formation (Benrimoh et al., 2018; Corlett et al., 2019; Parr et al., 2018). When coding Rorschach responses, most contemporary systems for use differentiate several levels to designate the quality with which percepts fit the inkblots at the location being used, known as Form Quality, including conventional or ordinary, unusual or idiosyncratic, and distorted or minus (e.g., Meyer & Mihura, 2021). Rorschach (1921/2021) noted that to produce responses with good Form Quality, respondents needed stable attention, clarity in their efforts at perceptual and associative integration, and self-control. As such, among his patients with schizophrenia, only those with paranoia produced reasonably conventional responses, while those with disorganized symptoms had a higher frequency of distorted or idiosyncratic perceptions. These observations by Rorschach have received consistent support in the subsequent research literature, which indicates Form Quality is an excellent marker of perceptual deviance and one of the best validated measures derived from the Rorschach (Meyer & Mihura, 2021; Mihura et al., 2013).

Rorschach research bearing on these issues that could inform an active inference model of perception supports the notion that unique perceptions can be associated with unduly weighted priors and insufficient regard for corrective environmental sensory feedback. Asari and colleagues (2008, 2010a, 2010b) conducted three interrelated studies of Form Quality scores that provide an understanding of the psychological operations active when a respondent is generating a response with particular types of Form Quality. The authors used functional and structural MRI to examine the neurophysiological features associated with atypical and distorted perceptions, uncommon perceptions, and conventional perceptions. A key finding was that in people giving atypical and distorted perceptions amygdala activity generated a positive, excitatory link between the right temporal pole and the left anterior prefrontal cortex, while simultaneously generating a negative, inhibitory effective connectivity from the right temporopolar region to the bilateral occipitotemporal regions.

Thus, atypical and distorted perceptions in this study involved instances when internal processes triggered by something in the inkblots activated affectively charged brain structures to turn off the typical process of reciprocal visual calibration between ideas and perceptual stimuli in favor of idiosyncratic, nonconsensual top–down views. In essence, sensory signals were shut down in favor of overly precise charged beliefs. Rather than taking in the visual cues the environment was providing, personally relevant, emotionally salient unique perceptions forced themselves into an inkblot representation, overriding the respondent's ability to perceive experiences in a conventional manner.

Concluding Comments

With this essay, we hope to have interested readers in the richly productive and increasingly broad literature on active inference and the Bayesian brain. In some depth, we outlined aspects of the evolutionary, biological, and neurophysiological foundation for this mathematically inspired model of functioning. We also identified psychologically relevant areas of active research that readers may find useful for further exploration and we closed by offering a handful of ways that Rorschach responding appears to fit seamlessly and meaningfully within an actively inferring Bayesian brain.

References

Adams, R. A., Brown, H. R., & Friston, K. J. (2014). Bayesian inference, predictive coding and delusions. *AVANT: The Journal of the Philosophical-Interdisciplinary Vanguard, V*(3), 51–88. https://doi.org/10.26913/50302014.0112.0004

Adams, R. A., Stephan, K. E., Brown, H. R., Frith, C. D., & Friston, K. J. (2013). The computational anatomy of psychosis. *Frontiers in Psychiatry, 4*, Article 47. https://doi.org/10.3389/fpsyt.2013.00047

Aggelopoulos, N. C. (2015). Perceptual inference. *Neuroscience and Biobehavioral Reviews, 55*, 375–392. https://doi.org/10.1016/j.neubiorev.2015.05.001

Akavia, N. (2013). *Subjectivity in motion: Life, art, and movement in the work of Hermann Rorschach (2012–34295-000)*. Routledge/Taylor & Francis Group.

Asari, T., Konishi, S., Jimura, K., Chikazoe, J., Nakamura, N., & Miyashita, Y. (2008). Right temporopolar activation associated with unique perception. *NeuroImage, 41*(1), 145–152. https://doi.org/10.1016/j.neuroimage.2008.01.059

Asari, T., Konishi, S., Jimura, K., Chikazoe, J., Nakamura, N., & Miyashita, Y. (2010a). Amygdalar enlargement associated with unique perception. *Cortex, 46*(1), 94–99. https://doi.org/10.1016/j.cortex.2008.08.001

Asari, T., Konishi, S., Jimura, K., Chikazoe, J., Nakamura, N., & Miyashita, Y. (2010b). Amygdalar modulation of frontotemporal connectivity during the inkblot test. *Psychiatry Research: Neuroimaging, 182*(2), 103–110. https://doi.org/10.1016/j.pscychresns.2010.01.002

Barrett, L. F. (2017). The theory of constructed emotion: An active inference account of interoception and categorization. *Social Cognitive and Affective Neuroscience, 12*(11), Article 1833. https://doi.org/10.1093/scan/nsx060

Benrimoh, D., Parr, T., Vincent, P., Adams, R. A., & Friston, K. (2018). Active inference and auditory hallucinations. *Computational Psychiatry (Cambridge, Mass.), 2*, 183–204. https://doi.org/10.1162/cpsy_a_00022

Berry, B. A., & Meyer, G. J. (2019). Contemporary data on the location of response objects in Rorschach's inkblots. *Journal of Personality Assessment, 101*(4), 402–413. https://doi.org/10.1080/00223891.2017.1408016

Brown, H., Adams, R. A., Parees, I., Edwards, M., & Friston, K. (2013). Active inference, sensory attenuation and illusions. *Cognitive Processing, 14*(4), 411–427. https://doi.org/10.1007/s10339-013-0571-3

Carhart-Harris, R. L. (2018). The entropic brain – Revisited. *Neuropharmacology, 142*, 167–178. https://doi.org/10.1016/j.neuropharm.2018.03.010

Carhart-Harris, R. L., & Friston, K. J. (2010). The default-mode, ego-functions and free-energy: A neurobiological account of Freudian ideas. *Brain: A Journal of Neurology, 133*(4), 1265–1283. https://doi.org/10.1093/brain/awq010

Clark, A. (2013). Whatever next? Predictive brains, situated agents, and the future of cognitive science. *Behavioral and Brain Sciences, 36*(3), 181–204. https://doi.org/10.1017/S0140525X12000477

Clark, A. (2016). *Surfing uncertainty: Prediction, action, and the embodied mind.* Oxford University Press.

Corlett, P. R., Horga, G., Fletcher, P. C., Alderson-Day, B., Schmack, K., & Powers, A. R. I. (2019). Hallucinations and strong priors. *Trends in Cognitive Sciences, 23*(2), 114–127. https://doi.org/10.1016/j.tics.2018.12.001

Davey, C. G., Pujol, J., & Harrison, B. J. (2016). Mapping the self in the brain's default mode network. *NeuroImage, 132*, 390–397. https://doi.org/10.1016/j.neuroimage.2016.02.022

Exner, J. E. (2003). *The Rorschach: A comprehensive system* (4th ed. Vol. 1). Wiley.

Exner, J. E. (1996). Critical bits and the Rorschach response process. *Journal of Personality Assessment, 67*(3), 464–477. https://doi.org/10.1207/s15327752jpa6703_3

Friston, K. (2009). The free-energy principle: A rough guide to the brain? *Trends in Cognitive Sciences, 13*(7), 293–301. https://doi.org/10.1016/j.tics.2009.04.005

Friston, K. (2013). Life as we know it. *Journal of The Royal Society Interface, 10*(86), Article 20130475. https://doi.org/10.1098/rsif.2013.0475

Friston, K., Adams, R. A., Perrinet, L., & Breakspear, M. (2012). Perceptions as hypotheses: Saccades as experiments. *Frontiers in Psychology, 3*, Article 151. https://doi.org/10.3389/fpsyg.2012.00151

Friston, K., Brown, H. R., Siemerkus, J., & Stephan, K. E. (2016). The dysconnection hypothesis (2016). *Schizophrenia Research, 176*(2–3), 83–94. https://doi.org/10.1016/j.schres.2016.07.014

Friston, K., Mattout, J., & Kilner, J. (2011). Action understanding and active inference. *Biological Cybernetics, 104*(1–2), 137–160. https://doi.org/10.1007/s00422-011-0424-z

Gigerenzer, G., & Hoffrage, U. (1995). How to improve Bayesian reasoning without instruction: Frequency formats. *Psychological Review, 102*(4), 684–704. https://doi.org/10.1037/0033-295X.102.4.684

Giromini, L., Viglione, D. J. Jr., Pineda, J. A., Porcelli, P., Hubbard, D., Zennaro, A., & Cauda, F. (2019). Human movement responses to the Rorschach and mirroring activity: An fMRI study. *Assessment, 26*(1), 56–69. https://doi.org/10.1177/1073191117731813

Giromini, L., Viglione, D. J., Zennaro, A., & Cauda, F. (2017). Neural activity during production of Rorschach responses: An fMRI study. *Psychiatry Research: Neuroimaging, 262*, 25–31. https://doi.org/10.1016/j.pscychresns.2017.02.001

Hohwy, J. (2016). The self-evidencing brain. *Noûs, 50*(2), 259–285. https://doi.org/10.1111/nous.12062

Kilner, J. M., Friston, K. J., & Frith, C. D. (2007). Predictive coding: An account of the mirror neuron system. *Cognitive Processing, 8*(3), 159–166. https://doi.org/10.1007/s10339-007-0170-2

Linson, A., Parr, T., & Friston, K. J. (2020). Active inference, stressors, and psychological trauma: A neuroethological model of (mal)adaptive explore-exploit dynamics in ecological context. *Behavioural Brain Research, 380*, Article 112421. https://doi.org/10.1016/j.bbr.2019.112421

Martin, J.-R., & Pacherie, E. (2019). Alterations of agency in hypnosis: A new predictive coding model. *Psychological Review, 126*(1), 133–152. https://doi.org/10.1037/rev0000134

Meyer, G. J., & Mihura, J. L. (2021). Rorschach Performance Assessment System (R-PAS) for assessing disordered thought and perception. In I. B. Weiner & J. H. Kleiger (Eds.), *Psychological assessment of disordered thinking and perception* (pp. 151–168). American Psychological Association. https://doi.org/10.1037/0000245-010

Meyer, G. J., Viglione, D. J., Mihura, J. L., Erard, R. E., & Erdberg, P. (2011). *Rorschach Performance Assessment System: Administration, coding, interpretation, and technical manual*. Rorschach Performance Assessment System LLC.

Mihura, J. L., Meyer, G. J., Dumitrascu, N., & Bombel, G. (2013). The validity of individual Rorschach variables: Systematic reviews and meta-analyses of the Comprehensive System. *Psychological Bulletin, 139*(3), 548–605. https://doi.org/10.1037/a0029406

Momenian-Schneider, S. H., Brabender, V. M., & Nath, S. R. (2009). Psychophysiological reactions to the response phase of the Rorschach and 16PF. *Journal of Personality Assessment, 91*(5), 494–496. https://doi.org/10.1080/00223890903088727

Newmark, C. S., Hetzel, W., & Frerking, R. A. (1974). The effects of personality tests on state and trait anxiety. *Journal of Personality Assessment, 38*(1), 17–20. https://doi.org/10.1080/00223891.1974.10119934

Newmark, C. S., Wheeler, D., Newmark, L., & Stabler, B. (1975). Test-induced anxiety with children. *Journal of Personality Assessment, 39*(4), 409–413. https://doi.org/10.1207/s15327752jpa3904_15

Otten, M., Seth, A. K., & Pinto, Y. (2017). A social Bayesian brain: How social knowledge can shape visual perception. *Brain and Cognition, 112*, 69–77. https://doi.org/10.1016/j.bandc.2016.05.002

Palmer, C. J., Lawson, R. P., & Hohwy, J. (2017). Bayesian approaches to autism: Towards volatility, action, and behavior. *Psychological Bulletin, 143*(5), 521–542. https://doi.org/10.1037/bul0000097

Parr, T., Benrimoh, D. A., Vincent, P., & Friston, K. J. (2018). Precision and false perceptual inference. *Frontiers in Integrative Neuroscience, 12*. https://doi.org/10.3389/fnint.2018.00039

Parr, T., & Friston, K. J. (2017). The active construction of the visual world. *Neuropsychologia, 104*, 92–101. https://doi.org/10.1016/j.neuropsychologia.2017.08.003

Parr, T., Pezzulo, G., & Friston, K. J. (2022). *Active inference: The free energy principle in mind, brain, and behavior*. MIT Press.

Rorschach, H. (2021). *Hermann Rorschach's psychodiagnostics: Newly translated and annotated 100th anniversary edition* (P. J. Keddy, R. Signer, P. Erdberg, & A. Schneider-Stocking, Eds. & Trans.). Hogrefe Publishing. (Original work published 1921)

Searls, D. (2017). *The inkblots: Hermann Rorschach, his iconic test, and the power of seeing*. Crown.

Seth, A. K. (2013). Interoceptive inference, emotion, and the embodied self. *Trends in Cognitive Sciences, 17*(11), 565–573. https://doi.org/10.1016/j.tics.2013.09.007

Solms, M., & Friston, K. (2018). How and why consciousness arises: Some considerations from physics and physiology. *Journal of Consciousness Studies, 25*(5–6), 202–238.

Villemor-Amaral, A. E., Yazigi, L., Nascimento, R. S. G. F., Primi, R., & Semer, N. L. (2007, July 25–28). *Localização, Qualidade Formal e Respostas Populares do Rorschach no SC em uma Amostra Brasileira* [Location, form quality and popular responses in the Rorschach CS in a Brazilian sample] [Paper presentation]. III Congresso Brasileiro de Avaliação Psicológica, João Pessoa, PB, Brasil. https://www.ibapnet.org.br/congresso2007/LivroMesas2007.pdf

Wiese, W., & Metzinger, T. K. (2017). Vanilla PP for philosophers: A primer on predictive processing. In T. Metzinger & W. Wiese (Eds.), *Philosophy and predictive processing: 1.* MIND Group. https://doi.org/10.15502/9783958573024

Zhou, Y., Friston, K. J., Zeidman, P., Chen, J., Li, S., & Razi, A. (2018). The hierarchical organization of the default, dorsal attention and salience networks in adolescents and young adults. *Cerebral Cortex, 28*(2), 726–737. https://doi.org/10.1093/cercor/bhx307

History
Received July 7, 2022
Revision received July 11, 2022
Accepted July 15, 2022
Published online September 2, 2022

Acknowledgments
We thank Daniel Collerton and the editor for their helpful recommendations on a previous version of this article. We are also grateful to Odile Hussain, Harald Janson, Ernesto Pais, and Tomoko Muramatsu for their help with the translation of the summary.

Conflict of Interest
The first author declares a potential conflict of interest in that he is a member of a company that sells products related to the Rorschach Performance Assessment System, which is indirectly referenced in this work. The second author declares no potential conflict of interest.

Gregory J. Meyer
Department of Psychology
University of Toledo
2925 W. Bancroft Street
Toledo, OH 43606
USA
gregory.meyer@utoledo.edu

Summary

In this review, we consider the Rorschach from the perspective of the brain processes that drive perceptual inference. We begin with a broad overview of Bayesian active inference, which postulates that all living organisms must maintain separateness from their environment in order to avoid entropic dissipation and non-sustaining environmental states. Organisms achieve these aims by generating *perceptions* that are the best hypothesis to explain their sensory impressions or by taking some *action* to better sample the environment in order to update perceptions. Perceptions are thus beliefs founded on Bayesian probabilities, which are updated as the top-down predictions encounter bottom-up contradictory sensory data that returns an error signal to be reconciled. The constant back and forth communication between prediction and error, as well as the required belief updating process rests sensitively upon the confidence ascribed to sensory input, relative to the confidence placed in prior beliefs about the causes of sensations. Predictions can be quite rudimentary, though for sentient organisms they are embedded in a neural hierarchy permitting a high degree of complexity and a capacity to envision alternative futures, which brings to the organism choice and agency. Active inference, with its focus on the balance between sensory precision and prior precision, is grounded in rigorously defined mathematical formalisms that are tightly linked to biologically plausible mechanisms of action. Active inference has advanced the science of artificial intelligence, robotics, neurophysiology, cognition (e.g., attention), interoception, and neuropsychology (e.g., false inference in hallucinations). For instance, false inference generally results from abnormally high precision afforded to high-level explanations for visual input, which may compensate for a failure to attenuate sensory precision. Given this, the Rorschach task provides an interesting paradigm because the amount of precise information about the causes of visual input is deliberately minimized – and rendered ambiguous – thereby placing greater emphasis on the respondent's prior beliefs. We thus consider how an active inference model of the mind meshes both with Rorschach's own views of the task, how it works, and what it provides, and with emerging neuroscience documenting the operations engaged by responding to the task. In particular, we note how Rorschach saw the task as one that slowed the normal process of visual perception to make the individual's apparatus for experiencing the environment visible to an assessor. We close by exploring three other Rorschach processes that seamlessly integrate with active inference, including envisioning human action, introversiveness and motility, and perceptual distortions.

Résumé

Dans cet article, nous envisageons le Rorschach du point de vue des processus cérébraux qui propulsent l'inférence perceptuelle. Nous commençons par un aperçu global de l'inférence active bayésienne, qui postule que tous les organismes vivants doivent maintenir une séparation de leur environnement, afin d'éviter la dissipation entropique et des états environnementaux insoutenables. Les organismes atteignent ces objectifs en générant des perceptions qui représentent alors la meilleure hypothèse pour expliquer leurs impressions sensorielles, ou en procédant à quelque action visant à mieux échantillonner l'environnement afin de mettre à jour leurs perceptions. Les perceptions sont donc des croyances fondées sur des probabilités bayésiennes, qui sont mises à jour au fur et à mesure que les prédictions descendantes rencontrent des données sensorielles ascendantes contradictoires qui renvoient un signal d'erreur à rectifier. L'oscillation permanente entre prédiction et erreur, ainsi que le processus nécessaire de mise à jour des croyances, s'appuient de manière sensible sur la confiance accordée à l'entrée sensorielle, elle-même liée à la confiance placée dans les croyances antérieures concernant les causes des sensations. Ces prédictions peuvent être assez rudimentaires; néanmoins chez les organismes sensibles, elles sont intégrées dans une hiérarchie neuronale permettant un haut degré de complexité ainsi qu'une capacité à envisager des futurs alternatifs, ce qui apporte à l'organisme choix et l'agence. L'inférence active, avec sa centration sur l'équilibre entre précision sensorielle et précision antérieure, est ancrée dans des formalismes mathématiques rigoureusement définis, qui sont intimement liés aux mécanismes d'action biologiquement plausibles. L'inférence active a avancé la science de l'intelligence artificielle, la robotique, la neurophysiologie, la science cognitive (par exemple, l'étude de l'attention), l'intéroception et la neuropsychologie (par exemple, la fausse inférence dans les hallucinations). Par exemple, la fausse inférence résulte généralement d'une précision anormalement élevée accordée aux explications de haut niveau de l'entrée visuelle et peut compenser l'échec d'une atténuation de la précision sensorielle. Compte tenu de cela, la tâche Rorschach fournit un paradigme intéressant, du fait qu'elle minimise délibérément la quantité d'informations précises sur les causes de l'entrée visuelle – en même temps qu'elle les rend ambiguës – mettant ainsi davantage l'accent sur les croyances antérieures du répondant. Nous considérons donc qu'un modèle de l'esprit d'inférence active s'intègre à la fois avec les vues de Rorschach lui-même sur la tâche, son fonctionnement et ce qu'elle permet, et avec la recherche émergente en neurosciences sur les opérations qui sont impliquées lors du processus de la réponse. En particulier, nous relevons comment Rorschach considérait la tâche comme ralentissant le processus normal de perception visuelle, permettant ainsi de rendre visible à un expérimentateur l'appareil d'un individu en train d'expérimenter l'environnement. Nous terminons en explorant trois autres processus Rorschach qui s'intègrent insensiblement à l'inférence active, notamment la représentation de l'action humaine, l'introversion et la motilité, et les distorsions perceptives.

Resumen

En este repaso, consideramos al Rorschach desde la perspectiva de los procesos cerebrales que impulsan la inferencia perceptiva. Comenzamos con una descripción general amplia de la inferencia activa Bayesiana en sus múltiples manifestaciones, la cual postula que todos los organismos vivos deben mantenerse separados de su entorno para evitar la disipación entrópica y los estados ambientales no sostenibles. Los organismos logran estos objetivos generando percepciones, que son la mejor hipótesis para explicar sus impresiones sensoriales, o tomando alguna acción para lograr mejores muestras del entorno con el fin de actualizar dichas percepciones. Estas últimas son, por lo tanto, creencias basadas en probabilidades Bayesianas, que se actualizan a medida que las predicciones top-down se encuentran con datos sensoriales bottom-up contradictorios que devuelven una señal de error que debe ser resuelta. La constante comunicación de ida y vuelta entre la predicción y el error, así como el proceso de actualización de creencias requerido, descansa sensiblemente sobre la confianza atribuida al input sensorial, relacionado con la confianza depositada en creencias previas sobre las causas de las sensaciones. Las predicciones pueden ser bastante rudimentarias, aunque para los organismos sensibles están integradas en una jerarquía neuronal que permite un alto grado de complejidad y una capacidad para visualizar futuros alternativos, lo que aporta al organismo posibilidad de elección y agencia. La inferencia activa, con su enfoque en el equilibrio entre las precisiones sensoriales y previas, se basa en formalismos matemáticos rigurosamente definidos que están estrechamente vinculados a mecanismos de acción biológicamente plausibles. La inferencia activa ha permitido avances en la inteligencia artificial, robótica, neurofisiología, cognición (por ejemplo, atención), interocepción y neuropsicología (por ejemplo, inferencia falsa en las alucinaciones). Por ejemplo, la inferencia falsa generalmente resulta de una inusualmente alta precisión otorgada a explicaciones de alto nivel para el input visual, lo que puede compensar una falla en la atenuación de la precisión sensorial. Dado esto, la tarea del Rorschach proporciona un paradigma interesante porque la cantidad de información precisa sobre las causas del input visual se minimiza deliberadamente -y se vuelve ambigua-, lo que pone mayor énfasis en las creencias previas de la persona evaluada. Por lo tanto, consideramos cómo un modelo de inferencia activa de la mente encuadra tanto con los propios puntos de vista de Rorschach sobre la tarea, cómo funciona y qué produce, así como también con la incipiente investigación neurocientífica que ha dado cuenta de las operaciones relacionadas con responder a la tarea. En particular, notamos cómo Rorschach vio la tarea como aquella que ralentizaba el proceso normal de percepción visual para hacer que el aparato del individuo que experimenta el entorno fuera visible para un evaluador.
    Cerramos explorando otros tres procesos del Rorschach que se integran a la perfección con la inferencia activa, incluida la visualización de la acción humana, introversión y movimiento, y las distorsiones perceptivas.

要約

このレビューでは、ロールシャッハを、知覚推論を惹起する脳プロセスの観点から考察する。まず、ベイズ型能動推論を概観すると、全ての生物はエントロピーの散逸と環境の非持続的状態を避けるために、環境からの分離性を維持していると仮定している。生物は、自分の感覚的印象を説明するのに最適な仮説である知覚を生成するか、知覚を更新するために環境をよりよくサンプリングするために何らかの行動を起こすことで、これらの目的を達成する。このように、知覚はベイズ推論の確立に基づく信念であり、トップダウンの予測がボトムアップの矛盾する感覚データに遭遇し、エラーシグナルを返すことで更新され、調整される。予測と誤りの間の絶え間ない往復運動と、必要な信念の更新プロセスは、感覚入力に与えられた信頼と、感覚の原因に関する事前の信念に置かれた信頼とに敏感に依存する。予測は非常に初歩的なものであるが、知覚を持つ生物にとっては、高度な複雑性と代替的な未来を想定する能力を可能にする神経階層に組み込まれており、それによって生物に選択と主体性がもたらされる。感覚的な正確さと事前の正確さのバランスに焦点を当てた能動的推論は、厳密に定義された数学的形式に基づいており、生物学的に妥当な作用機序と密接に結びついている。能動的推論は、人工知能、ロボット工学、神経生理学、認知（注意など）、相互知覚、神経心理学（幻覚の誤推論など）の科学を発展させた。例えば、一般に誤認識は、視覚入力に対する高次の説明に与えられる精度が異常に高く、感覚の精度を減衰させることの失敗を補うために生じることがある。ロールシャッハ課題では、信念を形成するための視覚的入力の正確な情報を意図的に限定し、曖昧にすることで回答者の事前確信がより強調されるため、興味深いパラダイムと言える。そこで、心の能動的推論モデルが、ロールシャッハ自身の課題に対する見解、課題の仕組み、課題から得られるもの、課題への反応に関わる操作を記録した新しい神経科学の両方とどのように噛み合うかを検討する。特に、ロールシャッハがこの課題が評価者に可視化するために通常の視覚的知覚のプロセスからその経験の認知に至るプロセスをゆっくり起こさせるものだと考えていたことに注目する。最後に、積極的な推論とシームレスに統合されるロールシャッハの他の3つのプロセス、すなわち、人間の行動の想像、内向性と運動性、知覚の歪みについて探求することによって締めくくる。

Special Issue: New Insights From Other Psychological Disciplines
for Rorschach Users
Original Article

The Right Hemisphere and Ambiguity

A Possible Role of Handedness in Rorschach Responsivity

Stephen Christman

Department of Psychology, University of Toledo, OH, USA

Abstract: The Rorschach Test has evolved from an idiosyncratic projective personality test to an evidence-based performance test used widely in forensic settings. The current paper argues that Rorschach researchers should consider the role of two related neuropsychological factors in the assessment of Rorschach responding: the role of the right cerebral hemisphere in the perception of ambiguous figures and the role of individual differences (as a function of consistency of handedness) in responding to ambiguous stimuli. The right hemisphere is more fluent and flexible in the perception of ambiguous stimuli. Moreover, individuals with mixed/inconsistent hand preference have greater access to right hemisphere processing, and, accordingly, are more fluent and flexible in their perception of ambiguous stimuli. This raises the possibility of quantitative and qualitative differences in Rorschach responsivity as a function of test takers' handedness. Implications of the presence of higher rates of schizotypy in inconsistent-handers are also discussed.

Keywords: Rorschach inkblot, individual differences, handedness, ambiguous figure perception, cerebral hemispheres

The Rorschach inkblot test has a long and storied history in the field of psychology and is enjoying a renaissance in the form of the emerging Rorschach Performance Assessment System (R-PAS) framework for administration and interpretation (e.g., Mihura & Meyer, 2018). As noted by Exner (1994), the Rorschach has proven effective at differentiating various groups: patients versus non-patients, patients with schizophrenia versus those with depression, etc. Exner goes on to stress that the Rorschach has potential utility as a measure of individual, not just group, differences, and he suggests that the use of the Rorschach Test as a measure of individual differences, "seems to be neglected most often by those using the test, and that neglect probably limits the quality of treatment offered to those who have been subjects of the test" (Exner, 1994, p. 7).

This neglect that Exner lamented persists, and the current article offers a new perspective on individual differences in Rorschach responsivity. To illustrate, PsycInfo searches were performed (on August 12, 2021) for six common psychological tests, three from the clinical realm (Rorschach, Minnesota Multiphasic Personality Inventory [MMPI], and the Thematic Apperception Test [TAT]) and three from the cognitive realm (Stroop test, Digit Span, and Wisconsin Card Sorting Test [WCST]). For each term, the total number of PsycInfo hits was recorded. Then, again for each term, the percentage of hits that also included one of the following search terms were also calculated: "individual differences," "sex differences," and "handedness." The results are presented in Table 1.

Inspection of Table 1 reveals some interesting features. The Rorschach has fewer results with "individual difference" and "sex" results than the other two clinical tests. Also, while the three cognitive tests have slightly higher percentages than the clinical tests for "individual differences," the clinical tests have slightly higher percentages for "sex differences." Most importantly, the cognitive tests are almost 30 times more likely than the clinical tests to return results for "handedness." Clearly, handedness is a neglected dimension of interest in much clinical work, and the purpose of this paper is to encourage Rorschach researchers in particular, and clinicians in general, to pay closer attention to potential handedness effects in their data sets. Interestingly, Rorschach explicitly chose to use symmetrical stimuli to avoid potential handedness difference in response biases (Sergent & Binik, 1979).

There are two lines of neuropsychological research that strongly suggest that handedness may be an important factor in Rorschach responsivity: (a) neuropsychological studies of brain activity while viewing inkblots indicating a special role of the right cerebral hemisphere, and (b) a growing body of research indicating that inconsistent-handedness is associated with greater access to right hemisphere processing and, hence, greater cognitive flexibility in dealing with ambiguity. Each of these lines of research will be reviewed in turn.

Neuropsychology of Inkblot Viewing

A number of brain imaging studies indicate greater right than left hemisphere activation while viewing inkblot stimuli. Hirotoshi et al. (2012) used near-infrared spectroscopy to look at prefrontal activation while participants viewed the pictorial stimuli from the Rorschach Inkblot Test, the Rozenzweig Picture-Frustration Study, and the TAT. Both the Rorschach and the TAT were associated with increased right prefrontal activation. By contrast, the Picture-Frustration Study stimuli were associated with increased left prefrontal activation, likely due in part to the fact that the stimuli include verbal captions, unlike the nonverbal stimuli used in the Rorschach and TAT. Using electroencephalographic (EEG) data, Gill

Table 1. PsycInfo results for common psychological tests as a function of individual difference searches

Primary search term	# Hits	% with "individual differences"	% with "sex differences"	% with "handedness"
Clinical tests				
Rorschach	11253	1.38	1.92	0.09
MMPI	12755	1.83	3.91	0.06
TAT	3471	2.62	4.00	0.09
Cognitive tests				
Stroop task	16481	4.42	1.61	2.36
Digit span	7481	4.48	2.17	1.95
WCST	8413	2.42	1.28	2.50

Note. MMPI = Minnesota Multiphasic Personality Inventory; TAT = Thematic Apperception Test; WCST = Wisconsin Card Sort Test.

and O'Boyle (2003) also reported greater right frontal activation while viewing inkblots, along with bilateral parietal and occipital activation.

Asari et al. (2008) studied functional magnetic resonance imaging (fMRI) responses while participants described what inkblot stimuli looked like. They found that right temporal lobe activation was associated with the production of unique responses, while left frontal and bilateral occipitotemporal activation was associated with typical responses.

Using fMRI data, Ishibashi et al. (2016) found increased right temporal activation, along with bilateral parietal and occipital activation when viewing achromatic inkblots. Interestingly, chromatic inkblots were associated with increased left hemisphere activation. This may reflect the fact that the colored regions in inkblots are localized to specific areas of the overall inkblot, and the left hemisphere is specialized for the processing of local levels of form, in contrast to the right hemisphere's specialization for processing global/holistic levels of form (Sergent, 1982; Van Kleeck, 1989). It should be noted that other imaging studies using inkblot stimuli fail to find lateralized effects, reporting bilateral activation across broad cortical regions (Giromini et al., 2016, 2019).

In a study comparing brain activation in normal controls versus patients with schizophrenia while describing inkblot stimuli, Kircher et al. (2002) reported that the amount of speech produced in the normal controls correlated mainly with left hemisphere activation, whereas in the patient group the correlation was mostly with right hemisphere activation. This suggests that the role of the right hemisphere in inkblot perception is enhanced in schizophrenia, which is important given that the Rorschach is often administered in forensic contexts to individuals with severe mental illness.

Further evidence for right hemisphere involvement in Rorschach perception comes from patient studies. Henninger (1996) presented inkblot stimuli to the left and right hemispheres of two split-brain patients and asked them to draw what they had seen, using the left hand for right hemisphere trials and the right hand for left hemisphere trials. Compared to right hemisphere trials, the drawing produced by the left hemisphere tended to be unidentifiable or to simply resemble the patients' verbal descriptions. The author concludes that the left hemisphere has difficulty with ambiguous shapes that cannot be verbally labelled.

Regard and Landis (1997) discuss an unpublished study on left versus right hemisphere inkblot responses in split-brain patients that found that the patients' responses to centrally presented inkblots were more similar to their left, relative to right, hemisphere responses, suggesting that standard administration of the Rorschach may not fully access right hemisphere mentation.

Finally, Lewis (1979) administered the Rorschach to eight split-brain patients and found that disconnection of the hemispheres led to increased perplexity (as measured by Piotrowski's Pix index, an "organic sign" of disordered brain function) and tended to destroy creativity, as measured by the M, W, and O+ scores on the Rorschach. As consistent-handers have lesser interhemispheric connectivity than inconsistent-handers (Luders et al., 2010), this result may have implications for handedness differences in Rorschach responsivity.

Hall and colleagues (1968) presented inkblot stimuli to patients with left versus right hemisphere lesions and found that right hemisphere lesions (and hence left hemisphere responding) were associated with incongruity between percept and blot and with inappropriate combinations of parts and whole with bizarre and preposterous results. This finding is another reflection of the importance of right hemisphere global processing in the ability to develop coherent interpretations of the entire blot.

In a similar study, Vilkki (1987) found that patients with left hemisphere damage had poor ideational productivity, whereas patients with right hemisphere damage had a perceptual disturbance indicated by a high number of diffuse color responses to whole blots. A study by Birch and Belmont (1961) of only patients with left hemisphere damage found that they showed lowered response productivity and increased acceptance of the stimulus as a whole and a decreased ability to reorganize the stimulus in terms of its parts, a finding again consistent with the right hemisphere's specialization for processing global, not local, levels of form.

By contrast, Gainotti et al. (1984) also administered Rorschach stimuli to patients with unilateral lesions and found no relationship between hemispheric lateral lesions and the type of Rorschach responses. These results from unilateral lesion studies are not very consistent, likely due in part to unassessed variations in the intrahemispheric location of lesions (and, particularly, the extent to which language areas in the left hemisphere were affected).

An unpublished study discussed by Regard and Landis (1997) involved participants taking the Holtzman Inkblot Test before and after left versus right medial temporal lobectomy. Left versus right hemisphere damage was associated with increased negativity (i.e., fear) versus positivity (i.e., joy) of emotional reactions to the inkblots. This finding likely reflects Davidson's work showing that the left versus right hemispheres are specialized for approach- versus withdrawal-related emotions, respectively (Davidson, 1993). Given evidence for greater risk (and hence withdrawal) sensitivity in inconsistent-handers (Christman, Jasper, et al., 2007), this suggests that the responses of inconsistent-handers may feature greater negative emotional content.

A study of patients with left versus right hemisphere benign (gliomas and meningiomas) tumors found that tumors of the right hemisphere were associated with fewer responses with precise form and an increased number of confabulatory interpretations with poor form, while left frontal tumors were associated with an overall reduction in the amount of responding (Belyi, 1983). Tumor studies have to be interpreted differently than lesion studies, as lesions are associated with decreased/absent activity in the affected brain area, while tumors are often associated with abnormal activation of affected brain areas (think of Charles Whitman, the University of Texas at Austin belltower sniper, and the tumor in his amygdala). From this perspective, the results of this tumor study suggest that the left hemisphere may generate fewer inkblot responses than the right hemisphere.

Behavioral studies with normal participants also point to a special role of the right hemisphere in inkblot responsivity. In a study by Minor and colleagues (1989), prior to viewing inkblot stimuli presented to the left or right visual field, participants heard two words, one describing an interpretation of the inkblot based on shape or form and one describing an interpretation based on chromatic color. They found the left hemisphere was biased toward color choices, while the right was biased toward form choices, echoing the neuroimaging results of Ishibashi et al. (2016). They conclude that the left hemisphere's favored mode of mental representation is semantic (e.g., choosing concepts associated with the names of colors in the inkblots), while the right hemisphere's favored representation is imaginal (e.g., choosing concepts associated with difficult-to-label forms in the inkblots).

Of particular relevance to the current paper are a pair of studies by Brugger and colleagues. Brugger et al. (1993) presented random dot patterns to the left and right visual fields and found a more pronounced readiness to see meaningful information when the dot pattern was presented to the left of fixation. In a follow-up study, Brugger and Regard (1995) presented inkblot stimuli to the left and right visual fields and again reported a consistent right hemisphere bias in seeing meaningful configurations in unstructured visual stimuli.

To provide a rough summary of the preceding literature review: (a) greater relative right hemisphere activation is found during administration of inkblot stimuli, especially in patients with schizophrenia; (b) the left hemisphere has particular problems processing ambiguous shapes that cannot be readily verbalized; (c) the left hemisphere is more sensitive to color while the right is more sensitive to form; (d) the right hemisphere generates more unique responses to inkblot stimuli; and (e) central administration of inkblots yields patterns of responding that are more reflective of left than right hemisphere responsivity.

Handedness, the Right Hemisphere, and Ambiguity

We are now ready to turn to handedness. Inconsistent-handedness is associated with greater functional access to right hemisphere processes (Prichard et al., 2013). This greater right hemisphere access is presumed to arise, at least in part, from the facts that (a) inconsistent-handedness is associated with larger corpus callosum size (Luders et al., 2010), and (b) inconsistent-handedness is associated with greater baseline levels of right hemisphere activation (Propper et al., 2012). Thus, given the importance of right hemisphere processing in inkblot responsivity, one would predict a difference between inconsistent- versus consistent-handers in performance on the Rorschach.

It is important to first specify what is meant by consistent- versus inconsistent-handedness. Our laboratory assesses handedness using the Edinburgh Handedness Inventory (EHI; Oldfield, 1971). It asks about 10 manual activities and responding is done on a 5-point scale (*always left, usually left, no preference, usually right, always right*), and yields scores ranging from −100 (perfect left-handedness) to +100 (perfect right-handedness). A median split done on the absolute value of EHI scores typically yields a median score of +80 (we use absolute values to collapse across degree of handedness). A score of +80 is equivalent to a person indicating that they do nine of the 10 activities always with the same hand but do the 10th with their other hand; "inconsistent-handed" does not connote ambidextrous. Thus, instead of the traditional 90%–10% split between right-handers and left-handers, we propose a 50%–50% split in the human population between consistent- and inconsistent-handers (Christman & Prichard, 2016).

A growing body of evidence suggests degree of handedness (consistent/strong vs. inconsistent/mixed) is a more fundamental dimension of human individual difference than is direction of handedness (right vs. left); see Prichard et al.,

2013, for a review. Inconsistent handedness is associated with greater baseline right hemisphere EEG activation (Propper et al., 2012), greater access to right frontal areas involved in episodic memory retrieval (Christman & Propper, 2010), greater access to right parietal areas involved in body image representation (Christman, Bentle, et al., 2007), and greater sensitivity to risk, which is mediated in part by right frontal areas (Christman, Jasper, et al., 2007).

The behavioral evidence for greater access to right hemisphere processing in inconsistent-handers has been interpreted in relation to the finding that the corpus callosum is appreciably larger in inconsistent-handers than in consistent right- or consistent left-handers (Luders et al., 2010), thus enabling greater interhemispheric interaction and right hemisphere access in inconsistent-handers.

Inconsistent-handedness is also associated with increased cognitive flexibility. For example, relative to consistent-handers, inconsistent-handers exhibit greater openness to experience (Bryson et al., 2009), decreased need for closure (Lyle & Grillo, 2020), greater openness to obscure musical genres (Christman, 2013), greater gullibility and openness to persuasion (Christman et al., 2008), increased tendency to update beliefs (Jasper et al., 2014), increased sensation seeking (Christman, 2014), greater flexibility in making consumer price decisions (Barone et al., 2015), greater fluency in dealing with ambiguous figures (Christman et al., 2009), greater appreciation of logical paradoxes (Niebauer & Garvey, 2004), increased divergent thinking (Shobe et al., 2009), a broader spread of semantic activation (Sontam & Christman, 2012), increased semantic switching during a verbal fluency task (Sontam et al., 2009), increased ability to take other people's perspectives into account (Rose et al., 2012; Lanning et al., in press), greater tolerance of uncertainty and ambiguity (Kumar et al., 2020), and decreased right-wing authoritarianism (Chan, 2018; Christman, 2014; Lyle & Grillo, 2014).

Generally speaking, inconsistent-hand preference is associated with greater tolerance of ambiguity, and greater ability at updating mental representations and holding contradictory representations at the same time. Thus, there are both neuropsychological (e.g., greater RH activation and greater RH access) and behavioral (greater cognitive flexibility and tolerance of ambiguity) reasons why inconsistent-handers may approach and react to the ambiguity of the Rorschach Test differently from consistent-handers.

Of central relevance to this point is a study by Christman et al. (2009). Experiments 1 and 2 presented participants with a series of images that gradually morphed from one object (e.g., a duck) into another (e.g., a rabbit), with the middle item in each series corresponding to a classic bistable ambiguous figure and asked them to name what they saw for each image. Inconsistent-handers updated to the second object earlier than consistent-handers. Experiment 3 was especially relevant: Participants were presented with various bistable ambiguous figures (e.g., the Necker Cube, the duck/rabbit figure) and inkblot stimuli for 60 s each and were asked to press a key each time their interpretation of the figure changed. This spontaneous reversal rate was much higher in inconsistent-handers: For the bistable figures, inconsistent-handers averaged about 21 reversals in the 60-s interval while consistent-handers average only about 12 reversals. For inkblot stimuli, the number of interpretation changes was smaller, but the same pattern of handedness difference was observed: about seven inkblot interpretations from inconsistent-handers over the 60-s viewing period, compared with only about three interpretations for consistent-handers.

Given that standard R-PAS protocols allow two to three interpretations per inkblot, the above results suggest that the range of potential Rorschach responsivity is being under-sampled in inconsistent-handers relative to consistent-handers. While R-PAS scoring is based more on *how* a person responds rather than on *what* they see in the inkblots, it is possible that the greater number of interpretations offered by inconsistent-handers may be associated with changes over time in how they respond.

While the results of both the handedness study by Christman et al. (2009) and the visual half-field study by Brugger and Regard (1995) addressed only quantitative differences (more interpretations by inconsistent-handers, more interpretations by the right hemisphere), it is likely that there are qualitative differences as well between inconsistent- and consistent-handers (and between left and right hemisphere presentations), given the role of the right hemisphere in Rorschach responsivity and the fact that inconsistent-handers have greater right hemisphere access.

The author is aware of only one study that looked at qualitative differences as a function of handedness in Rorschach responsivity. Finn and Neuringer (1968) reported that left-handers gave significantly more White Space responses than right-handers, and interpreted this as reflecting greater oppositional tendencies in left-handers. It is not clear, however, how this finding relates to the current framework.

There are a few more data about qualitative hemispheric differences in Rorschach responsivity, summarized in a review by Regard and Landis (1997). Regard et al. (1985) presented Rorschach plates to the left and right visual fields, and found that there were significantly more F+ and combinatory responses (D-W, W2, CF+F) and more M and O- to left visual field/right hemisphere stimulation while there were more W1, F-, and FC and more rejections to right visual field/left hemisphere presentations. "Psychograms" constructed by a trained Rorschach practitioner for each hemisphere contrasted in interesting ways: The right hemisphere was better able to combine and synthesize form elements, more intuitive, and more affectively toned, while the left hemisphere lacked spontaneity, was more dry and tedious but also fairly well-adjusted.

Maurer (1990) presented inkblots to the left and right visual fields and asked normal participants to indicate how much they liked or disliked each stimulus. There were no visual field differences observed. Regard (1991) conducted a similar study with split-brain patients and again found no hemispheric differences in response valence. However, it is not clear how much the "liking" or "disliking" of Rorschach stimuli is relevant to the R-PAS system.

Implications for Individual Differences in Rorschach Responding

So, what does this all mean for Rorschach Test users? One possibility involves the use of norms in the R-PAS: Just as there have been separate norms for children versus adolescents versus adults, perhaps there should also be different norms for consistent- versus inconsistent-handers. Of particular relevance to this point is the finding that central administration of inkblots yields patterns of responding that are more reflective of left than right hemisphere responsivity. This finding is likely more reflective of consistent-handers' responsivity, given inconsistent-handers' greater functional access to right hemisphere processes; perhaps inconsistent-handers yield more right hemisphere-like patterns of responding.

A related issue concerns how well R-PAS norms work across different cultures. Raymond and Pontier (2004) reported left-handedness rates for various countries. They found a wide range of left-handedness rates, from a low of 6.4% in Japan to a high of 23.2% in France. While there are no data on national differences in rates of consistency of handedness, left-handedness rates can be used as a rough proxy for inconsistent-handedness rates, as the majority of left-handers are inconsistent handed (Christman & Prichard, 2016; Prichard et al., 2013). To the extent that the Rorschach responsivity of consistent- versus inconsistent-handers is indeed different, then one might expect different norms for countries with very low versus high rates of left-/inconsistent-handedness.

Another potentially relevant issue involves the fact that inconsistent-handers generate more interpretations of Rorschach stimuli than do consistent-handers (Christman et al., 2009). This suggests that the range of possible Rorschach responsivity in inconsistent-handers is being under-sampled. Future work may want to look at if and how Rorschach responsivity changes over multiple interpretations (beyond the two currently allowed in the R-PAS protocol) of a given Rorschach plate.

A hint as to specific ways that inconsistent- versus consistent-handers may differ in Rorschach responsivity can be found in the results of Burin et al. (2019). They looked at relations between Rorschach responsivity and susceptibility to the "rubber-hand illusion," finding that increased susceptibility was positively with the Perception and Thinking Problems and Self and Other Presentation domains. Given evidence that inconsistent-handers are more susceptible to the rubber-hand illusion (Niebauer et al., 2002), perhaps inconsistent-handers' responsivity is also positively correlated with those two Rorschach domains.

Similarly, Petot (2005) reported that increased Openness to Experience was related to Rorschach low L, high blends, morbid responses, and combinatory special scores. They also established that response style does not moderate correlations between Openness and the Rorschach. Given evidence that inconsistent-handedness is associated with increased Openness to Experience (Bryson et al., 2009), perhaps inconsistent-handedness is also related to those Rorschach variables.

One last relevant issue concerns the fact that inconsistent-handedness is a reliable predictor of both schizotypy (e.g., Somers et al., 2009; Tran et al., 2015) and schizophrenia (e.g., Dragovic & Hammond, 2005; Sommer et al., 2001). Given that the Rorschach is often administered in forensic situations and/or to persons with severe mental illness, it is possible that inconsistent-handedness is over-represented among Rorschach samples. If so, this would highlight the importance of establishing different norms for inconsistent- versus consistent-handed individuals, as it may be difficult to distinguish between aspects of Rorschach responsivity that reflect normal right hemisphere forms of responding versus pathological forms of responding.

When Hermann Rorschach first developed his inkblots, he explicitly chose to use symmetrical stimuli, as he feared asymmetrical stimuli would be treated differently by left- versus right-handed individuals (Sergent & Binik, 1979). It is a bit ironic that his choice of ambiguous stimuli means that his test may be treated differently by inconsistent- versus consistent-handed individuals.

References

Asari, T., Konishi, S., Jimura, K., Chikazoe, J., Nakamura, N., & Miyashita, Y. (2008). Right temporopolar activation associated with unique perception. *NeuroImage, 41*(1), 145–152. https://doi.org/10.1016/j.neuroimage.2008.01.059

Barone, M. B., Lyle, K. B., & Winterich, K. P. (2015). When deal depth doesn't matter: How handedness consistency influences consumer response to horizontal versus vertical price comparisons. *Marketing Letters, 26*(2), 213–223. https://doi.org/10.1007/s11002-013-9276-8

Belyi, B. I. (1983). Reflection of functional hemispheric asymmetry in some phenomena of visual perception. *Human Physiology, 8,* 410–417.

Birch, H. G., & Belmont, I. (1961). Functional levels of disturbance manifested by brain-damaged (left hemiplegic) patients as revealed in Rorschach responses. *Journal of Nervous and Mental Disease, 132*(5), 410–416. https://doi.org/10.1097/00005053-196105000-00005

Brugger, P., & Regard, M. (1995). Rorschach inkblots in the peripheral visual fields: Enhanced associative quality to the left of fixation. *Journal of Genetic Psychology, 156*(3), 385–387. https://doi.org/10.1080/00221325.1995.9914831

Brugger, P., Regard, M., Landis, T., Cook, N., Krebs, D., & Niederberger, J. (1993). "Meaningful" patterns in visual noise: Effects of lateral stimulation and the observer's belief in ESP. *Psychopathology, 26*(5–6), 261–265. https://doi.org/10.1159/000284831

Bryson, F. M., Grimshaw, G. M., & Wilson, M. S. (2009). The role of intellectual openness in the relationship between hand preference and positive schizotypy. *Laterality, 14*(5), 441–456. https://doi.org/10.1080/13576500802349684

Burin, D., Pignolo, C., Ales, F., Giromini, L., Pyasik, M., Ghirardello, D., Zennaro, A., Angiletta, M., Castellino, L., & Pia, L. (2019). Relationships between personality features and the rubber hand illusion: An exploratory study. *Frontiers in Psychology, 10*, Article 2762. https://doi.org/10.3389/fpsyg.2019.02762

Chan, E. Y. (2018). Handedness and religious beliefs: Testing the two possible accounts of authoritarianism and belief updating. *Personality and Individual Differences, 127*, 101–106. https://doi.org/10.1016/j.paid.2018.02.005

Christman, S. D. (2013). Handedness and "earedness": Strong right-handers are less likely to prefer obscure musical genres. *Psychology of Music, 41*(1), 89–96. https://doi.org/10.1177/0305735611415751

Christman, S. D. (2014). Individual differences in personality as a function of degree of handedness: Consistent-handers are less sensation seeking, more authoritarian, and more sensitive to disgust. *Laterality, 17*, 354–367. https://doi.org/10.1080/1357650X.2013.838962

Christman, S. D., Bentle, M., & Niebauer, C. L. (2007). Handedness differences in body image distortion and eating disorder symptomatology. *International Journal of Eating Disorders, 40*, 247–256. https://doi.org/10.1002/eat.20357

Christman, S. D., Henning, B. R., Geers, A. L., Propper, R. E., & Niebauer, C. L. (2008). Mixed-handed persons are more easily persuaded and are more gullible: Interhemispheric interaction and belief updating. *Laterality, 13*(5), 403–426. https://doi.org/10.1080/13576500802079646

Christman, S. D., Jasper, J. D., Sontam, V., & Cooil, B. (2007). Individual differences in risk perception versus risk taking: Handedness and interhemispheric interaction. *Brain and Cognition, 63*(1), 51–58. https://doi.org/10.1016/j.bandc.2006.08.001

Christman, S. D., & Prichard, E. C. (2016). Half oaks, half willows: Degree, not direction, of handedness underlies both stable prevalence in the human population and species-beneficial variations in cognitive flexibility. *Evolutionary Psychological Science, 2*, 228–236. https://doi.org/10.1007/s40806-016-0047-7

Christman, S., & Propper, R. (2010). An interhemispheric basis for episodic memory: Effects of handedness and bilateral eye movements. In G. Davies & D. Wright (Eds.), *Current issues in applied memory* (pp. 185–205). Psychology Press.

Christman, S. D., Sontam, V., & Jasper, J. D. (2009). Individual differences in ambiguous figure perception: Degree of handedness and interhemispheric interaction. *perception, 38*, 1183–1198. https://doi.org/10.1068/p6131

Davidson, R. J. (1993). Cerebral asymmetry and emotion: Conceptual and methodological conundrums. *Cognition and Emotion, 7*, 115–138. https://doi.org/10.1080/02699939308409180

Dragovic, M., & Hammond, G. (2005). Handedness and schizophrenia: A quantitative review of evidence. *Acta Psychiatrica Scandinavica, 111*, 410–419. https://doi.org/10.1111/j.1600-0447.2005.00519.x

Exner, J. E. Jr. (1994). Rorschach and the study of the individual. *Rorschachiana, 19*(1), 7–23. https://doi.org/10.1027/1192-5604.19.1.7

Finn, J. A., & Neuringer, C. (1968). Left-handedness: A study of its relation to opposition. *Journal of Projective Techniques & Personality Assessment, 32*, 49–52. https://doi.org/10.1080/0091651X.1968.10120446

Gainotti, G., de Rosa, E., & Fischetti, C. (1984). Spécialisation hémisphérique et traitement analytique et gestaltique des informations. Une recherche avec le test de Rorschach [Hemispheric specialization and analytical and gestaltic processing of information. Research with the Rorschach Test]. *Revue de Psychologie Appliquée, 34*, 89–98.

Gill, H. S., & O'Boyle, M. (2003). Generating an image from an ambiguous visual input: An electroencephalographic (EEG) investigation. *Brain and Cognition, 51*, 287–293. https://doi.org/10.1016/S0278-2626(03)00032-0

Giromini, L., Viglione, D. J., Pineda, J., Porcelli, P., Hubbard, D., Zennaro, A., & Cauda, F. (2019). Human movement responses to the Rorschach and mirroring activity: An fMRI study. *Assessment, 26*, 56–69. https://doi.org/10.1177/1073191117731813

Giromini, L., Viglione, D. J., Zennara, A., & Cauda, F. (2016). Neural activity during production of Rorschach responses: An fMRI study. *Psychiatry Research: Neuroimaging, 262*, 25–31. https://doi.org/10.1016/j.pscychresns.2017.02.001

Hall, M. M., Hall, G. C., & Lavoie, P. (1968). Ideation in patients with unilateral or bilateral midline brain lesions. *Journal of Abnormal Psychology, 73*, 526–531. https://doi.org/10.1037/h0026515

Henninger, P. (1996). Inkblot testing of commisurotomy subjects: Contrasting modes of organizing reality. In S. Hameroff, A. W. Kaszniak, & A. C. Scott (Eds.), *Toward a science of consciousness: The first Tucson discussions and debates* (pp. 203–221). MIT Press.

Hirotoshi, H., Haida, M., Matsumoto, M., Hayakawa, N., Inomata, S., & Matsumoto, H. (2012). Differences of prefrontal cortex activity between picture-based personality tests: A near-infrared spectroscopy study. *Journal of Personality Assessment, 94*, 366–371. https://doi.org/10.1080/00223891.2012.666597

Ishibashi, M., Uchiumi, C., Jung, M., Aizawa, N., Makita, K., Nakamura, Y., & Saito, D. N. (2016). Difference in brain hemodynamics in response to achromatic and chromatic cards of the Rorschach: A fMRI study. *Rorschachiana, 37*(1), 41–57. https://doi.org/10.1027/1192-5604/a000076

Jasper, J. D., Kunzler, J., Prichard, E. C., & Christman, S. D. (2014). Individual differences in information order effects: The importance of right-hemisphere access in belief updating. *Acta Psychologica, 148*, 115–122. https://doi.org/10.1016/j.actpsy.2014.01.004

Kircher, T. T. J., Liddle, P. F., Brammer, M. J., Williams, S. C. R., Murray, R. M., & McGuire, P. K. (2002). Reversed lateralization of temporal activation during speech production in thought disordered patients with schizophrenia. *Psychological Medicine, 32*, 439–449. https://doi.org/10.1017/S0033291702005287

Kumar, S., Saini, R., & Jain, R. (2020). Hand preference and intolerance of uncertainty: Atypical cerebral lateralization advantages lower intolerance of uncertainty. *Laterality, 25*(1), 22–42. https://doi.org/10.1080/1357650X.2019.1611843

Lanning, M. D., Christman, S. D., & Fugget, A. (in press). Social comparison and handedness: Mixed handers are less susceptible to egocentric biases in judgments about others' performance. *Personality and Individual Differences*.

Lewis, R. T. (1979). Organic signs, creativity, and personality characteristics of patients following cerebral commissurotomy. *Clinical Neuropsychology, 1*, 29–33.

Lyle, K. B., & Grillo, M. C. (2014). Consistent-handed individuals are more authoritarian. *Laterality, 19*(2), 146–163. https://doi.org/10.1080/1357650X.2013.783044

Luders, E., Cherbuin, N., Thompson, P. M., Gutman, B., Anstey, K. J., Sachdev, P., & Toga, A. W. (2010). When more is less: Associations between corpus callosum size and handedness lateralization. *NeuroImage, 52*, 43–49. https://doi.org/10.1016/j.neuroimage.2010.04.016

Lyle, K. B., & Grillo, M. C. (2020). Why are consistently-handed individuals more authoritarian? The role of need for cognitive closure. *Laterality, 25*(4), 490–510. https://doi.org/10.1080/1357650X.2020.1765791

Maurer, A. (1990). *Preference and classification of emotional stimuli: A lateralized tachistoscopic experiment* (Diploma thesis). Seminar of Applied Psychology.

Mihura, J. L., & Meyer, G. J. (2018). Introduction to R-PAS. In J. L. Mihura & G. J. Meyer (Eds.), *Using the Rorschach Performance Assessment System (R-PAS)* (pp. 3–22). Guilford Press.

Minor, S. W., White, H., & Owings, E. P. (1989). Hemispheric asymmetries in interpreting forms vs colors in ambiguous patterns. *Brain and Cognition, 9*, 123–135. https://doi.org/10.1016/0278-2626(89)90048-1

Niebauer, C., Aselage, J., & Schutte, C. (2002). Interhemispheric interaction and consciousness: Degree of handedness predicts the intensity of a sensory illusion. *Laterality, 7*(1), 85–96. https://doi.org/10.1080/13576500143000159

Niebauer, C. L., & Garvey, K. (2004). Gödel, Escher, and degree of handedness: Differences in interhemispheric interaction predict differences in understanding self-reference. *Laterality, 9*(1), 19–34. https://doi.org/10.1080/13576500342000130

Oldfield, R. C. (1971). The assessment and analysis of handedness: The Edinburgh Inventory. *Neuropsychologia, 9*, 97–113. https://doi.org/10.1016/0028-3932(71)90067-4

Petot, J.-M. (2005). Are the relationships between NEO PI-R and Rorschach markers of openness to experience dependent on the patient's test-taking attitude? *Rorschachiana, 27*(1), 30–50. https://doi.org/10.1027/1192-5604.27.1.30

Prichard, E., Propper, R. E., & Christman, S. D. (2013). Degree of handedness, but not direction, is a systematic predictor of cognitive performance. *Frontiers in Psychology, 4*, 3–6. https://doi.org/10.3389/fpsyg.2013.00009

Propper, R. E., Pierce, J., Geisler, M. W., Christman, S. D., & Bellorado, N. (2012). Asymmetry in resting alpha activity: Effects of handedness. *Open Journal of Medical Psychology, 1*, 86–90. https://doi.org/10.4236/ojmp.2012.14014

Raymond, M., & Pontier, D. (2004). Is there geographical variation in human handedness? *Laterality, 9*(1), 35–52. https://doi.org/10.1080/13576500244000274

Regard, M. (1991). *The perception and control of emotion: Hemispheric differences and the role of the frontal lobes* (Habilitation thesis). University of Zürich.

Regard, M., & Landis, T. (1997). Hemispheric differences in the processing of ambiguity: Tachistoscopic studies with inkblots. *Rorschachiana, 22*(1), 114–129. https://doi.org/10.1027/1192-5604.22.1.114

Regard, M., Landis, T., & Bash, K. W. (1985). Affectivity: Tachistoscopic evidence of hemispheric differences. In F. Schmielau (Ed.), *Psychologie in der Medizin* (pp. 10–11). München.

Rose, J. P., Jasper, J. D., & Corser, R. (2012). Interhemispheric interaction and egocentrism: The role of handedness in social comparative judgement. *British Journal of Social Psychology, 51*, 111–129. https://doi.org/10.1111/j.2044-8309.2010.02007.x

Sergent, J. (1982). The cerebral balance of power: Confrontation or cooperation? *Journal of Experimental Psychology: Human Perception and Performance, 8*, 253–272. https://doi.org/10.1037/0096-1523.8.2.253

Sergent, J., & Binik, Y. M. (1979). On the use of symmetry in the Rorschach Test. *Journal of Personality Assessment, 43*, 355–359. https://doi.org/10.1207/s15327752jpa4304_3

Shobe, E. R., Ross, N. M., & Fleck, J. I. (2009). Influence of handedness and bilateral eye movements on creativity. *Brain and Cognition, 71*(3), 204–214. https://doi.org/10.1016/j.bandc.2009.08.017

Somers, M., Sommer, I. E., Boks, M. P., & Kahn, R. S. (2009). Hand-preference and population schizotypy: A meta-analysis. *Schizophrenia Research, 108*, 25–32. https://doi.org/10.1016/j.schres.2008.11.010

Sommer, I., Ramsey, N., Kahn, S., Aleman, A., & Bouma, A. (2001). Handedness, language lateralisation and anatomical asymmetry in schizophrenia: Meta-analysis. *British Journal of Psychiatry, 178*, 344–351. https://doi.org/10.1192/bjp.178.4.344

Sontam, V., & Christman, S. D. (2012). Semantic organization and handedness: Mixed-handedness is associated with more diffuse activation of ambiguous word associates. *Laterality, 17*(1), 38–50. https://doi.org/10.1080/1357650X.2010.529450

Sontam, V., Christman, S. D., & Jasper, J. D. (2009). Individual differences in semantic switching flexibility: Effects of handedness. *Journal of the International Neuropsychological Society, 15*, 1023–1027. https://doi.org/10.1017/S1355617709990440

Tran, U. S., Stieger, S., & Voracek, M. (2015). Mixed-footedness is a more relevant predictor of schizotypy than mixed-handedness. *Psychiatry Research, 225*, 446–451. https://doi.org/10.1016/j.psychres.2014.11.069

Van Kleeck, M. (1989). Hemispheric differences in global versus local processing of hierarchical visual stimuli by normal subjects: New data and a meta-analysis of previous studies. *Neuropsychologia, 27*, 1165–1178. https://doi.org/10.1016/0028-3932(89)90099-7

Vilkki, J. (1987). Ideation and memory in the inkblot technique after focal cerebral lesions. *Journal of Clinical and Experimental Neuropsychology, 9*, 699–710. https://doi.org/10.1080/01688638708405211

History
Received November 4, 2021
Revision received November 22, 2021
Accepted December 6, 2021
Published online August 10, 2022

Conflict of Interest
The author has no conflicts of interest to declare.

ORCID
Stephen Christman
https://orcid.org/0000-0003-1773-6332

Stephen Christman
Department of Psychology
University of Toledo
Toledo, OH 43606
USA
stephen.christman@utoledo.edu

Summary

Exner (1994) lamented the neglect of individual, as opposed to group, differences in the study and use of the Rorschach Inkblot Test. This neglect persists to this day, particularly in regard to individual differences as a function of degree (consistent vs. inconsistent) of handedness. Inconsistent-handedness is associated with increased access to right hemisphere processes, increased right hemisphere activation, and increased interhemispheric callosal connectivity. Moreover, inconsistent-handedness is also associated with greater cognitive flexibility and increased tolerance of ambiguity.

Brain imaging and patient studies are reviewed, revealing a special role of the right hemisphere during Rorschach responding: The right hemisphere generates more interpretations overall, more unique interpretations, and is more sensitive to form (while the left hemisphere is more sensitive to color). Also, responses to centrally presented inkblot stimuli more closely resemble left hemisphere responding than right hemisphere responding. The importance of the right hemisphere in Rorschach responsivity along with the greater access to right hemisphere processing in inconsistent-handers combine to suggest the potential existence of systematic differences as a function of degree of handedness.

Indeed, behavioral studies show greater flexibility and fluency in inconsistent-handers in generating meaningful interpretations of ambiguous stimuli, including inkblots. To date, only a handful of studies have looked at possible handedness differences in Rorschach responsivity, but (a) none have compared consistent- and inconsistent-handers and (b) none have been conducted within the R-PAS framework.

It is recommended that Rorschach researchers start paying attention to handedness effects in their data sets. It is possible that such handedness effects could be large enough to justify developing separate norms for the two handedness groups. Also, given large country-by-country variations in handedness rates, there could be a need to develop separate cultural/national norms. Finally, there is a strong association between inconsistent-handedness and both schizotypy and schizophrenia. Given that the Rorschach is often administered to populations with severe mental illness, it is possible that such data sets may contain a disproportionate number of inconsistent-handers, and it may be difficult to distinguish between aspects of Rorschach responsivity that reflect normal right hemisphere forms of responding versus pathological forms of responding.

Résumé

Exner (1994) a déploré la négligence des différences individuelles, par opposition au groupe, dans l'étude et l'utilisation du test de Rorschach Inkblot. Cette négligence persiste à ce jour, en particulier en ce qui concerne les différences individuelles en fonction du degré (cohérent contre inconsistant) de l'impartialité. Le manque de cohérence est associé à un accès accru aux processus de l'hémisphère droit, à une activation accrue de l'hémisphère droit et à une connectivité calleuse interhémisphérique accrue. De plus, l'inconstance est également associée à une plus grande flexibilité cognitive et à une tolérance accrue à l'ambiguïté.

L'imagerie cérébrale et les études de patients sont passées en revue, révélant un rôle particulier de l'hémisphère droit lors de la réponse de Rorschach : l'hémisphère droit génère globalement plus d'interprétations, plus d'interprétations uniques et est plus sensible à la forme (tandis que l'hémisphère gauche est plus sensible à la couleur). De plus, les réponses aux stimuli des taches d'encre présentés de manière centrale ressemblent plus à une réponse de l'hémisphère gauche qu'à une réponse de l'hémisphère droit. L'importance de l'hémisphère droit dans la réceptivité de Rorschach, ainsi que le plus grand accès au traitement de l'hémisphère droit chez les personnes inconsistantes, se combinent pour suggérer l'existence potentielle de différences systématiques en fonction du degré de maniabilité. En effet, les études comportementales montrent une plus grande flexibilité et une plus grande aisance chez les personnes inconsistantes pour générer des interprétations significatives de stimuli ambigus, y compris les taches d'encre. À ce jour, seule une petite poignée d'études ont examiné d'éventuelles différences de maniabilité dans la réactivité de Rorschach, mais (i) aucune n'a comparé les manieurs cohérents et incohérents et (ii) aucune n'a été menée dans le cadre du R-PAS.

Il est recommandé aux chercheurs de Rorschach de commencer à prêter attention aux effets de la latéralité dans leurs ensembles de données. Il est possible que de tels effets de latéralité soient suffisamment importants pour justifier l'élaboration de normes distinctes pour les deux groupes de latéralité. De plus, étant donné les grandes variations d'un pays à l'autre dans les taux d'utilisation manuelle, il pourrait être nécessaire de développer des normes culturelles/nationales distinctes.

Enfin, il existe une forte association entre l'inconstance et la schizotypie et la schizophrénie. Étant donné que le Rorschach est souvent administré à des populations atteintes de maladie mentale grave, il est possible que de tels ensembles de données contiennent un nombre disproportionné de personnes inconsistantes, et il peut être difficile de faire la distinction entre les aspects de la réactivité du Rorschach qui reflètent les formes normales de l'hémisphère droit. réponses versus formes pathologiques de réponse.

Resumen

Exner (1994) lamentó la negligencia de las diferencias individuales, a diferencia de las grupales, en el estudio y uso de la prueba de mancha de tinta de Rorschach. Esta negligencia persiste hasta el día de hoy, particularmente con respecto a las diferencias individuales en función del grado (consistente versus inconsistente) de destreza. La mano inconsistente se asocia con un mayor acceso a los procesos del hemisferio derecho, una mayor activación del hemisferio derecho y una mayor conectividad callosa interhemisférica. Además, la mano inconsistente también se asocia con una mayor flexibilidad cognitiva y una mayor tolerancia a la ambigüedad.

Se revisan las imágenes cerebrales y los estudios de pacientes, que revelan un papel especial del hemisferio derecho durante la respuesta de Rorschach: el hemisferio derecho genera más interpretaciones en general, más interpretaciones únicas y es más sensible a la forma (mientras que el hemisferio izquierdo es más sensible al color). Además, las respuestas a los estímulos de manchas de tinta presentadas centralmente se parecen más a la respuesta del hemisferio izquierdo que a la del hemisferio derecho. La importancia del hemisferio derecho en la capacidad de respuesta de Rorschach, junto con el mayor acceso al procesamiento del hemisferio derecho en manos inconsistentes, se combinan para sugerir la posible existencia de diferencias sistemáticas en función del grado de destreza manual. De hecho, los estudios del comportamiento muestran una mayor flexibilidad y fluidez en las manos inconsistentes para generar interpretaciones significativas de estímulos ambiguos, incluidas las manchas de tinta. Hasta la fecha, solo un pequeño puñado de estudios ha analizado las posibles diferencias de mano en la capacidad de respuesta de Rorschach, pero (i) ninguno ha comparado manos consistentes e inconsistentes y (ii) ninguno se ha realizado dentro del marco de R-PAS.

Se recomienda que los investigadores de Rorschach comiencen a prestar atención a los efectos de las manos en sus conjuntos de datos. Es posible que tales efectos de la mano derecha sean lo suficientemente grandes como para justificar el desarrollo de normas separadas para los grupos de las dos manos. Además, dadas las grandes variaciones de un país a otro en las tasas de uso de las manos, podría ser necesario desarrollar normas culturales / nacionales separadas.

Finalmente, existe una fuerte asociación entre la mano inconsistente y tanto la esquizotipia como la esquizofrenia. Dado que el Rorschach a menudo se administra a poblaciones con enfermedades mentales graves, es posible que dichos conjuntos de datos contengan un número desproporcionado de manos inconsistentes, y puede ser difícil distinguir entre aspectos de la capacidad de respuesta del Rorschach que reflejan formas normales del hemisferio derecho de responder versus formas patológicas de responder.

要約

Exner (1994)は、ロールシャッハ・インクブロット・テストの研究とその使用について、集団ではなく個人の差異を軽視していることを残念に思っていた。特に利き手の程度の個人差（一貫性のあるものと一貫性のないもの）に関して、個別性の軽視が現在も続いている。利き手が一貫していないことは、右半球のプロセスへの増加、右半球の活性化の増加、及び半球間の脳梁への接続の増加に関連している。さらに、一貫性のない利き手は、より大きな認定的柔軟性と曖昧さへの耐性の増加とも関連する。

　脳画像研究と症例研究をレビューし、ロールシャッハ反応における右半球の特別な役割を明らかにした。右半球は、全体的により多くの解釈をし、より多くのユニークな解釈を作り出し、そして形態についてより敏感である（一方、左半球は色に対してより敏感である）。また、中央に提示されたインクブロット刺激に対する反応は、右半球の反応よりも左半球の反応に近い。ロールシャッハ反応における右半球の重要性、及び、一貫性のない利き手では右半球処理にアクセスしやすいことから、利き手の程度による系統的な違いが存在する可能性が示唆される。

　実際、行動研究ではインクブロットなどの曖昧な刺激に対して、意味のある解釈を行う際、一貫性のない利き手を持つ方が、柔軟で流暢であることが示されている。これまで、ロールシャッハの応答性に見られる利き手の違いの可能性を検討した研究は僅かだが、(a) 一貫性のある利き手と一貫性のない利き手を比較したものはなく、(b) R-PASで実施されたものもなかった。

　ロールシャッハの研究者は、データセットにおける利き手の効果に注意を払い始めることが推奨される。このような利き手の効果は、2つの利き手グループに対して別々の基準（標準）を開発することを正当化するほど大きな可能性がある。また、利き手の比率が国よって大きく異なることから、文化的/国別標準を開発する必要があるかもしれない。最後に、一貫性のない利き手と統合失調型及び統合失調症の間には強い相関がある。ロールシャッハは重篤な精神疾患を持つ人々に実施されることが多いことを考えると、このようなデータセットには不釣り合いな数の一貫性のない利き手の持ち主が含まれる可能性があり、ロールシャッハへの反応性の側面が正常な右半球の反応様式と病的な反応様式を区別することが難しい場合もあるだろう。

Special Issue: New Insights From Other Psychological Disciplines
for Rorschach Users
Original Article

An Update on Social Touch

How Does Humans' Social Nature Emerge at the Periphery of the Body?

Elena Capelli[1], Serena Grumi[1], Eleonora Fullone[2],
Elisa Rinaldi[2], and Livio Provenzi[1]

[1]Child Neurology and Psychiatry Unit, IRCCS Mondino Foundation, Pavia, Italy
[2]Department of Brain and Behavioral Sciences, University of Pavia, Italy

Abstract: Recent research suggests that early physical touch provided by caregivers play a critical role in cognitive and affective development. The discovery of the C-tactile fibers – which selectively respond to low-speed physical stimulations, such as maternal affectionate touch and caresses – opened a promising field of research into the physiological bases of human togetherness. Notably, C-tactile fiber stimulation is primarily elaborated in a specific brain area (i.e., the insula), which is involved in affective and socio-cognitive skills as well as in the development of an individual's body image. In the present study, we provide a narrative overview of the research conducted so far on the role of maternal affectionate touch in infants' cognitive and emotional development, and we highlight potential implications for clinical practice with children and adults.

Keywords: C-tactile fibers, child development, parenting, social touch

The idea that our mind is rooted in the body is not new. Freud already suggested that the ego may ultimately derive from physical and bodily sensations originating from the body's surface (Freud, 1961). In the psychoanalytic field, Anzieu (1989) proposed to consider the ego-skin as a psychic envelope that enables specific mental functions such as containment, protection, delimitation, separation, and differentiation. Building on Anzieu's theoretical architecture, Werbart has proposed that the skin might be considered as the real cradle of our psyche (Werbart, 2019). Others have elaborated different theoretical assumptions that highlight the relevance of our body for our psychological development and functioning. In transactional analysis, the concept of positive and negative caresses is used to explain how relational transactions develop and affect our mental health (Berne, 1972). According to Berne, we transact with others by exchanging caresses. In the Rorschach inkblots test, texture responses are highly relevant for identifying individuals who might present abnormal management of their need for interpersonal contact and affective closeness (Cassella & Viglione, 2009), and they have

Rorschachiana (2022), 43(2), 168–185
https://doi.org/10.1027/1192-5604/a000153

been recently considered as a proxy for attachment assessment (Iwasa & Ogawa, 2013).

More recent advances at the intersection of neuroscience, psychology, and physiology are shedding new light on the mechanisms through which we are meant to be in touch, literally. The discovery of the social vestiges of the C-tactile fibers (McGlone et al., 2014) suggests that we may have a specialized and distributed neurophysiological network that signals social touch from the peripheral skin to the central nervous system. In this contribution, we provide an overview of social touch and C-tactile fibers and we highlight some implications in different contexts of human development and socio-affective functioning. A developmental framework is adopted here by focusing on the study of early social touch interactions to provide readers with a rationale on the foundational role of interpersonal contact for human psychology.

Beyond the Supremacy of Vision

Human social interactions are largely studied in scientific psychology. Nonetheless, this field has usually focused on how humans process visual social stimuli. Facial expression dynamics are a key feature of human social interactions (Jack & Schyns, 2015) through which humans display a wide range of emotional states and intentional cues. Moreover, it has been suggested that our ability to communicate and share emotions and intentions through facial expressions is deeply linked with evolutionarily sculpted mechanisms of neurophysiological stress regulation, providing us with an integrated and socially adapted psychophysiological system to deal with everyday challenges (Porges, 2007). As such, it is not surprising that facial expressions are highly relevant signals from the very beginning of life.

Three-month-old infants are facilitated in face recognition tasks when positive emotional expressions are shown by adults (Turati et al., 2011). Seven-month-old infants are already capable of using gaze information from complex face stimuli in rule-extraction tasks (Bulf et al., 2015). Nonetheless, during the first months of life, infants not only acquire relevant socio-cognitive knowledge about conspecifics' faces, but they also rapidly become specialized in analyzing and attributing meanings to specific hand movements. For instance, newborns in their first day of life look longer toward an impossible hand movement compared to a possible one (Longhi et al., 2015). At 6 months, they show anticipatory eye movements toward observed goal-directed actions (Falck-Ytter et al., 2006). Finally, head-mounted camera studies have shown that, after a precocious period of face supremacy in their visual field, hands become the primary target of attention as infants get older (Fausey et al., 2016).

Indeed, from birth, infants are naturally exposed to a constant stream of interconnected social–communicative signals that include face expressions, hand gestures but also speech, and interpersonal touch (Abu-Zhaya et al., 2016). The relevance of nonvisual social cues is even more evident in the case of developmental conditions in which the access to visual stimuli is reduced, for example, in infants with visual impairments. These infants may be less responsive to parents' communications in face-to-face and play interactions, yet they might still be capable of using their parents' behavioral inputs (e.g., turn-taking, parental sensitivity) to achieve adaptive socio-emotional and cognitive outcomes (Grumi et al., 2021). Thus, at least part of our communicative exchanges passes through sensory modalities other than visual cues, such as interpersonal touch.

Social Touch as a Key Component of Human Social Interactions

Animal model research suggests that social touch is involved in neural circuits maturation, executive functions improvement, and social development (Simpson et al., 2019). In rats, the quality of early maternal caregiving largely relies on physical contact. Behaviors such as licking, grooming, and arched-back nursing are highly influential on the maturation and development of the pups (Bagot et al., 2012). Male rats raised by high-contact dams are less reactive to stress, are better explorers in new environments, and have better learning and memory outcomes (Liu et al., 1997). More recently, maternal contact in mice significantly modulated pups' brain activity in the anterior cingulate cortex (Courtiol et al., 2018).

Is it possible that social touch – a behavioral exchange at the periphery of our bodies – is embedded into offspring's biology and contributes to shape developmental programming? Recent behavioral epigenetics research has provided a fascinating response to this question (Meaney & Szyf, 2005). Rat pups from mothers who expressed high-quality caregiving – characterized by high levels of licking and grooming – showed altered profiles of DNA expression in specific stress-related genes. These environmental-driven alterations in DNA transcriptional activity and gene expression may be mediated by epigenetic mechanisms, such as DNA methylation, that are highly susceptible to environmental stimulations, including caregiving behaviors (Provenzi, Brambilla, et al., 2020). In humans, the quality of maternal touch – even in the presence of severe postnatal maternal depression – has been found to be protective for infants' behavioral development

(Sharp et al., 2012). These effects are at least partially mediated by epigenetic mechanisms occurring in stress-related genes, such as the *SLC6A4* (Provenzi et al., 2016) or the *NR3C1* genes (Berretta et al., 2021).

Of course, social touch, and caregiving in general, is far more complex in humans compared to rodents. Studying the quality of early mother–infant interactions, Stack and colleagues (Jean et al., 2009) have largely documented many different types of maternal touch, which differ for cinematic features and functions. Depressed mothers might specifically avoid affective, playful, and stimulatory touch when regulating their infants' distress (Mantis et al., 2014). Moreover, a similar variability has also been documented in the way infants intentionally produce tactile stimulations directed toward the caregiver (Moszkowski et al., 2009), further highlighting the complexity of our social touch interactions from the very beginning of life. More recently, maternal social touch has been found to affect orienting of attention in children with disabilities, suggesting that the key role of tactile components of human relationships is not secondary even when atypical conditions are present (Provenzi, Rosa, et al., 2020).

From the Skin to the Brain

Social touch is today one of the most important royal roads to understanding the social nature of humans. Nonetheless, to fully understand the potential of social touch it is necessary to understand where and how it is elaborated in our central nervous system. Among the diverse touch modalities, energic and rhythmic tactile stimulations are often associated with playful interactions, whereas gentle stroking by individuals with whom we share an intimate affective bonding is usually associated with feelings of affiliations and pleasant response (Suvilehto et al., 2015). Gentle touch – typical of caresses and maternal touch with newborns and infants – when applied on the hairy skin specifically activates a response from a class of unmyelinated fibers, namely, the C-tactile fibers (Löken et al., 2009). Cutaneous C-tactile fibers are a vast and heterogenous population of unmyelinated, slowly conducting nerves, that potentially evolved to provide basic protective functions such as detecting and transmitting information of negatively (e.g., nociceptive) and positively (e.g., affection) hedonic events from the skin of the body or viscera to the brain (McGlone et al., 2014). These fibers respond to both pleasant and painful stimuli and have an early maturation. They are responsive to pain in preterm infants from 25 postconceptional weeks (Slater et al., 2006). Like adults, children show a clear preference for tactile stimulations that activate the C-tactile fibers (Croy et al., 2019) and electroencephalographic (EEG) evidence of the C-tactile system response to gentle stroking has been observed in infants as young as 11–36 days (Tuulari et al., 2019). The optimal firing response of C-tactile fibers has been found to be elicited by stroking at 1–10 cm/s (Löken et al., 2009), the same speed of self-reported pleasant perception of social touch, measured psychophysically (Essick et al., 2010). As such, they are meant to play a key role in encoding socio-affective and rewarding dimensions of interpersonal physical contact (McGlone et al., 2014).

The posterior insular cortex is a primary cortical target for C-tactile fibers (Björnsdotter et al., 2009). A recent study found that selective lesions in the posterior and anterior right insula significantly impact the perceived affectivity of C-tactile optimal touch, which results in a reduction of pleasantness sensitivity in its perception (Kirsch et al., 2020). It has recently been suggested that the brain network that elaborates pleasant social touch extends from the posterior insula to other brain regions involved in socio-emotional and socio-cognitive processing. These include the posterior superior temporal sulcus, the medial prefrontal cortex, the amygdala, the orbitofrontal cortex, and the dorsal anterior cingulate cortex (Olausson et al., 2010). Not surprisingly, these same regions are largely involved in both maternal (Bjertrup et al., 2019) and paternal (Provenzi et al., 2021) brain sensitivity to infant-related static and dynamic stimuli, further suggesting that the brain network that underpins social touch is embedded into a wider caregiving brain network.

Social touch is not merely a mechanical event; rather, it is a key component of human affective exchanges from infancy to adulthood, it evolved to serve adaptive advantage, and relies on brain networks that are deeply involved in the early parent–child interaction (Cascio et al., 2019). In the next paragraphs, we will provide examples of how social touch is involved in many different domains of human functioning across development and in adult life.

Social Touch Throughout Human Development

Body Ownership and Self–Other Discrimination

It is within the early parent–infant interactive dance that the self–other differentiation emerges during the first months of life. While visual stimuli have been previously hypothesized to serve a pivotal role in infants' capacity for self–other discrimination (Rochat, 2021), Montirosso and McGlone (2020) have highlighted the role played by social affectionate touch in the early emergence of body ownership and self–other differentiation. According to an embodied social-cognition approach, the authors provide a systematic account of recent evidence on the role played by low-pace C-tactile-like touch in the precocious behavioral markers of rudimentary distinctions between infants' own bodies and the external environment. Filippetti and colleagues (2013) have measured the looking behavior of newborns who were facing visuo-tactile synchronous or asynchronous stimuli. In both conditions, the newborns' face was stroked using a paintbrush every 10 s, while the newborns watched previously videotaped clips of a 5-month-old infant being brushed in the same way, synchronously or asynchronously. The synchronous and asynchronous trials were alternated, and the order of presentation, as well as the cheek on which the infant was brushed, was counterbalanced across infants. Infants showed a marked preference for synchronous presentations. In a subsequent study, newborns were also capable of discriminating among different loci of spatial congruence between the observed and the experienced touch occurrences (Filippetti et al., 2015). Starting from this evidence and considering that the affectionate touch style of parents is relatively stable across infancy (Mercuri et al., 2019), Montirosso and McGlone (2020) have hypothesized that parents are active contributors to their infants' sense of body ownership and self-other differentiation, and that they do so by engaging in reciprocal bodily contacts.

Socio-Affective Development and Emotional Regulation

Parental social touch may also provide a critical source of caregiving support to infants' emotional regulation and socio-affective development. Jean and colleagues' research (2009) on parent–infant reciprocal touch has suggested that different touch modalities are observed very early in life: playful touch, a very active, playful, dynamic, repetitive, and fast-paced tactile stimulation oriented at making the infant smile and laugh; attention-getting touch, such as tapping, patting, squeezing, and other tactile stimulations aimed at orienting the attention of the infant to the mother or the environment; finally, gentle or nurturing touch, a soothing and slow tactile stimulation, such as stroking and massaging. When infants are exposed to socio-emotional stress, mothers make greater use of nurturing touch to calm and regulate infants' behavior. At the same time, developmental risk conditions – such as preterm birth (Jean & Stack, 2012) and maternal depression (Mercuri et al., 2019) – seem to alter the early socio-tactile caregiving environment with negative consequences for infants' emotional regulation.

Cognitive Development

Social touch can affect different domains of cognitive development, including attention, executive functions, inhibitory control, and object exploration. First, maternal touch is beneficial for infants' learning. Four-month-old infants previously habituated to an individual averted-gaze face – which is typically not interesting for them – were able to recognize and discriminate these stimuli when parents provided low-speed stroking, but not when they were exposed to the task without tactile support (Della Longa et al., 2019). This study suggests that social touch can also affect child cognitive development. Not surprisingly, Tanaka and colleagues (2018) found that the brain activity of 8-month-old infants in response to pseudo-words was higher for the stimuli previously introduced with a multi-sensory training (audio and tactile stimulations) compared to sound-only control stimuli. Coherently, Seidl and colleagues (2015) reported that 4-month-old infants performed better in a task of speech-segmentation and word-finding when tactile cues were provided synchronously with the acoustic ones. Six-to-eight-month-old infants from dyads characterized by high-frequency physical contact exhibit greater object exploration compared to peers from dyads characterized by less physical contact (Tanaka et al., 2021). Even later in life, preschool children are more able to wait for a reward in the famous "marshmallow task" when the request to wait is accompanied by a friendly touch on the back (Leonard et al., 2014).

When Touch Is Challenged

Not only touch itself but also its absence can have a relevant effect on infants' development when adverse developmental conditions are present. Preterm infants who are hospitalized in the neonatal intensive care unit (NICU) are exposed to a stressful environment that is characterized by high-frequency pain and a partial absence of nurturing caregiver touch (Montirosso & Provenzi, 2015). Not surprisingly, even in absence of severe medical comorbidities, these infants are at heightened risk for developmental problems such as neurological conditions, sensorial deficits, as well as cognitive and emotional disorders (Stoll et al., 2010). Nonetheless, the adverse effects of the altered socio-tactile NICU environment can be reduced by interventions that maximize the precocious establishment of the physical and emotional intimate bonding between parents and their at-risk infant (Westrup, 2007). Skin-to-skin contact, the facilitation of maternal breastfeeding, and kangaroo care largely rely on parent–infant social touch and have beneficial impacts on preterm infants' outcomes and on parental mental health (Grundt et al., 2021). The promotion of social touch in the NICU improves the infant overall medical outcome and reduces the length of hospital stay (He et al., 2021). Moreover, parent-led skin-to-skin reduces infants' stress (Campbell-Yeo et al., 2019) and neuroendocrine reactivity to handling (Mörelius et al., 2015). Globally, skin-to-skin promotes better brain maturation (Scher et al., 2009) and neurobehavioral development, including short- and long-term psychomotor and cognitive indexes (Head, 2014).

Social Touch in Action in Adult Life

Romantic Attachment and Social Touch

In adults, affectionate touch is a powerful way to communicate intimacy and closeness. Not only is there evidence of C-tactile fiber activation in adults receiving touch during reciprocal stroking, but humans also tend to adjust the stroking velocity according to degrees of sympathy and interindividual attraction (Novembre, Etzi, & Morrison, 2021). It has been estimated that a romantic couple may spend 85% of the time in physical contact during a 4-hr period (Debrot et al., 2013). Additionally, love partners share the largest body surface allowed to be touched in social interactions. As the level of confidence and closeness between people decreases, the number of body areas available for physical contact also decreases, and the minimum number of areas is registered in the case of strangers (Suvilehto et al., 2015). Recent scientific literature also shows that social touch in romantic relationships plays a pivotal role in promoting personal well-being (Jakubiak & Feeney, 2017) and mental health with long-term effects (Debrot et al., 2021). In a functional magnetic resonance imaging (fMRI) task, oxytocin administration increased individuals' ratings of touch pleasantness when they assumed they were touched by their partner; moreover, in this condition heightened responses of the nucleus accumbens and anterior cingulate cortex were observed (Kreuder et al., 2017). Not surprisingly, it has been hypothesized that C-tactile afferents may act as mediators, at skin level, for oxytocin release, especially during affiliative tactile exchanges (Walker et al., 2017). In another fMRI study, holding hands with a romantic partner – compared to being alone – has been documented to reduce the reactivity of the anterior cingulate cortex and anterior insula while exposed to sadness-inducing pictures (Kraus et al., 2020).

Touch in Psychotherapy

Touch in psychotherapy has always been controversial. In Freud's earliest work, touch did not seem to be excluded, and there are indications of its use (Breuer & Freud, 1957). However, he quickly discouraged therapists on the use of physical contact with patients, and traditional psychoanalytic theories mainly valued the analyst's distance and the presence of clear physical boundaries with the patients by promoting the myth of the neutral analyst. In a large survey, almost 90% of psychotherapists declared they "never or rarely" actively touched clients, apart from a handshake at session beginnings or endings (Stenzel & Rupert, 2004). More recently, it has been suggested that forcibly eliminating physical contact from the therapeutic interaction can actively modify the relationship between patient and therapist, leading to further affective limitations to the dyadic exchange (Westland, 2011). The use of touch may be beneficial for specific patients, such as those who suffer from intense depersonalization symptoms after traumas (Fosshage, 2000) or patients with functional neurological symptoms associated with dissociative symptoms (Moenter, 2020). Some authors have also recently proposed the possibility of integrating therapeutic touch (e.g., massage) into a multidisciplinary approach for patients with affective disorders (Müller-Oerlinghausen & Eggart, 2021).

Touch Hunger During the COVID-19 Pandemic

At the time of writing, the world has been dramatically affected by the COVID-19 pandemic. Emotional distress and anxiety have been reported in medical staff (Barello et al., 2020) and patients (Vindegaard & Benros, 2020), but also in the general population (Giannopoulou et al., 2021). The pandemic has not only triggered a wide range of psychological symptoms mostly related to anxiety and depression, but it has also made seeking and receiving psychological support more difficult for people who experienced mental health difficulties (de Lima et al., 2020). Among the many stressing factors linked to the pandemic, social contact deprivation immediately became a worldwide issue as progressive and pervasive social-distancing measures have been adopted to mitigate and contain the virus spreading. As previously anticipated for preterm infants, the absence of social touch for prolonged periods can have a relevant and long-lasting psychosocial and neurobiological impact on human behavior and well-being. Moreover, the chronic lack of meaningful physical contact (e.g., touch hunger) has been previously shown to have a negative effect on mood, sleep, and overall physiological well-being in adults as well (Golaya, 2021). The metaphor of touch starvation (Durkin et al., 2021) has also been used in relation to the unprecedented suspension of social and physical contacts during the COVID-19 healthcare emergency. Isolation can have contributed through biological stress mechanisms to heightened risk of depression, anxiety, insomnia, and mental disorder exacerbation (Banerjee et al., 2021), as touch is involved in physiological and psychological processes linked to feelings of comfort, security, and satisfaction (Cascio et al., 2019).

Conclusion

Touch is a pervasive dimension of humans' social nature, and it permeates any relational exchange, from neonatal life to adulthood, from mother–infant bonding to romantic love. The recent advances in social neuroscience provide a reasonable rationale and a testable neurophysiological mechanism linking tactile stimulations occurring at the periphery of our body with key central neural processing involved in multisensory integration, emotion regulation, and cognitive functions. While the implications of this field are already translated into pragmatic actions in specific fields (e.g., preterm birth and skin-to-skin interventions), the broader impact of social touch neuroscience on human mental health is yet to be fully explored and determined (Croy et al., 2019). Nonetheless, while there is still much to be understood, it is already crystal clear that social touch – as a key dimension of human togetherness – cannot be left out of the room by researchers and health-care practitioners.

References

Abu-Zhaya, R., Seidl, A., & Cristia, A. (2016). Multimodal infant-directed communication: How caregivers combine tactile and linguistic cues. *Journal of Child Language, 44*(5), 1088–1116. https://doi.org/10.1017/S0305000916000416

Anzieu, D. (1989). *The skin ego.* Yale University Press.

Bagot, R. C., Zhang, T.-Y., Wen, X., Nguyen, T. T. T., Nguyen, H.-B., Diorio, J., Wong, T. P., & Meaney, M. J. (2012). Variations in postnatal maternal care and the epigenetic regulation of metabotropic glutamate receptor 1 expression and hippocampal function in the rat. *Proceedings of the National Academy of Sciences of the United States of America, 109*(Suppl 2), 17200–17207. https://doi.org/10.1073/pnas.1204599109

Banerjee, D., Vasquez, V., Pecchio, M., Hegde, M. L., Ks Jagannatha, R., & Rao, T. S. (2021). Biopsychosocial intersections of social/affective touch and psychiatry: Implications of "touch hunger" during COVID-19. *The International Journal of Social Psychiatry*, 20764021997485. https://doi.org/10.1177/0020764021997485

Barello, S., Palamenghi, L., & Graffigna, G. (2020). Burnout and somatic symptoms among frontline healthcare professionals at the peak of the Italian COVID-19 pandemic. *Psychiatry Research, 290.* https://doi.org/10.1016/j.psychres.2020.113129

Berne, E. (1972). *What do you say after you say hello? The psychology of human destiny.* Grove Press.

Berretta, E., Guida, E., Forni, D., & Provenzi, L. (2021). Glucocorticoid receptor gene (NR3C1) methylation during the first thousand days: Environmental exposures and developmental outcomes. *Neuroscience and Biobehavioural Reviews, 125*, 493–502. https://doi.org/10.1016/j.neubiorev.2021.03.003

Bjertrup, A. J., Friis, N. K., & Miskowiak, K. W. (2019). The maternal brain: Neural responses to infants in mothers with and without mood disorder. *Neuroscience and Biobehavioural Reviews, 107*, 196–207.

Björnsdotter, M., Löken, L., Olausson, H., Vallbo, Å., & Wessberg, J. (2009). Somatotopic organization of gentle touch processing in the posterior insular cortex. *Journal of Neuroscience, 29*(29), 9314–9320. https://doi.org/10.1523/JNEUROSCI.0400-09.2009

Breuer, J., & Freud, S. (1957). *Studies on hysteria.* Basic Books.

Bulf, H., Brenna, V., Valenza, E., Johnson, S. P., & Turati, C. (2015). Many faces, one rule: The role of perceptual expertise in infants' sequential rule learning. *Frontiers in Psychology, 6.* https://doi.org/10.3389/fpsyg.2015.01595

Campbell-Yeo, M., Johnston, C. C., Benoit, B., Disher, T., Caddell, K., Vincer, M., Walker, C.-D., Latimer, M., Streiner, D. L., & Inglis, D. (2019). Sustained efficacy of kangaroo care for repeated painful procedures over neonatal intensive care unit hospitalization: A single-blind randomized controlled trial. *Pain, 160*(11), 2580–2588. https://doi.org/10.1097/j.pain.0000000000001646

Cascio, C. J., Moore, D., & McGlone, F. (2019). Social touch and human development. *Developmental Cognitive Neuroscience, 35*, 5–11. https://doi.org/10.1016/j.dcn.2018.04.009

Cassella, M. J., & Viglione, D. J. (2009). The Rorschach texture response: A construct validation study using attachment theory. *Journal of Personality Assessment, 91*(6), 601–610. https://doi.org/10.1080/00223890903230931

Courtiol, E., Wilson, D. A., Shah, R., Sullivan, R. M., & Teixeira, C. M. (2018). Maternal regulation of pups' cortical activity: Role of serotonergic signaling. *ENeuro, 5*(4). https://doi.org/10.1523/ENEURO.0093-18.2018

Croy, I., Sehlstedt, I., Wasling, H. B., Ackerley, R., & Olausson, H. (2019). Gentle touch perception: From early childhood to adolescence. *Developmental Cognitive Neuroscience, 35*, 81–86. https://doi.org/10.1016/j.dcn.2017.07.009

de Lima, C. V. C., Cândido, E. L., da Silva, J. A., Albuquerque, L. V., de Soares, L. M., do Nascimento, M. M., de Oliveira, S. A., & Neto, M. L. R. (2020). Effects of quarantine on mental health of populations affected by Covid-19. *Journal of Affective Disorders, 275*, 253–254. https://doi.org/10.1016/j.jad.2020.06.063

Debrot, A., Schoebi, D., Perrez, M., & Horn, A. B. (2013). Touch as an interpersonal emotion regulation process in couples' daily lives: The mediating role of psychological intimacy. *Personality & Social Psychology Bulletin, 39*(10), 1373–1385. https://doi.org/10.1177/0146167213497592

Debrot, A., Stellar, J. E., MacDonald, G., Keltner, D., & Impett, E. A. (2021). Is touch in romantic relationships universally beneficial for psychological well-being? The role of attachment avoidance. *Personality & Social Psychology Bulletin, 47*(10), 1495–1509. https://doi.org/10.1177/0146167220977709

Della Longa, L., Gliga, T., & Farroni, T. (2019). Tune to touch: Affective touch enhances learning of face identity in 4-month-old infants. *Developmental Cognitive Neuroscience, 35*, 42–46. https://doi.org/10.1016/j.dcn.2017.11.002

Durkin, J., Jackson, D., & Usher, K. (2021). Touch in times of COVID-19: Touch hunger hurts. *Journal of Clinical Nursing, 30*(1–2), e4–e5. https://doi.org/10.1111/jocn.15488

Essick, G. K., McGlone, F., Dancer, C., Fabricant, D., Ragin, Y., Phillips, N., Jones, T., & Guest, S. (2010). Quantitative assessment of pleasant touch. *Neuroscience and Biobehavioural Reviews, 34*(2), 192–203. https://doi.org/10.1016/j.neubiorev.2009.02.003

Falck-Ytter, T., Gredebäck, G., & Von Hofsten, C. (2006). Infants predict other people's action goals. *Nature Neuroscience, 9*(7), 878–879. https://doi.org/10.1038/nn1729

Fausey, C. M., Jayaraman, S., & Smith, L. B. (2016). From faces to hands: Changing visual input in the first two years. *Cognition, 152*, 101–107. https://doi.org/10.1016/j.cognition.2016.03.005

Filippetti, M. L., Johnson, M. H., Lloyd-Fox, S., Dragovic, D., & Farroni, T. (2013). Body perception in newborns. *Current Biology, 23*(23), 2413–2416. https://doi.org/10.1016/j.cub.2013.10.017

Filippetti, M. L., Orioli, G., Johnson, M. H., & Farroni, T. (2015). Newborn body perception: Sensitivity to spatial congruency. *Infancy, 20*(4), 455–465. https://doi.org/10.1111/infa.12083

Fosshage, J. L. (2000). The meanings of touch in psychoanalysis: A time for reassessment. *Psychoanalytic Inquiry, 20*(1), 21–43. https://doi.org/10.1080/07351692009348873

Freud, S. (1961). *The ego and the id.* Norton.

Giannopoulou, I., Galinaki, S., Kollintza, E., Adamaki, M., Kympouropoulos, S., Alevyzakis, E., Tsamakis, K., Tsangaris, I., Spandidos, D. A., Siafakas, N., Zoumpourlis, V., & Rizos, E. (2021). COVID-19 and post-traumatic stress disorder: The perfect "storm" for mental health. *Experimental and Therapeutic Medicine, 22*(4), Article 1162. https://doi.org/10.3892/etm.2021.10596

Golaya, S. (2021). Touch-hunger: An unexplored consequence of the COVID-19 pandemic. *Indian Journal of Psychological Medicine, 43*(4), 362–363. https://doi.org/10.1177/02537176211014469

Grumi, S., Cappagli, G., Aprile, G., Mascherpa, E., Gori, M., Provenzi, L., & Signorini, S. (2021). Togetherness, beyond the eyes: A systematic review on the interaction between visually impaired children and their parents. *Infant Behaviour and Development, 64*, Article 101590. https://doi.org/10.1016/j.infbeh.2021.101590

Grundt, H., Tandberg, B. S., Flacking, R., Drageset, J., & Moen, A. (2021). Associations between single-family room care and breastfeeding rates in preterm infants. *Journal of Human Lactation: Official Journal of International Lactation Consultant Association, 37*(3), 593–602. https://doi.org/10.1177/0890334420962709

He, F. B., Axelin, A., Ahlqvist-Björkroth, S., Raiskila, S., Löyttyniemi, E., & Lehtonen, L. (2021). Effectiveness of the close collaboration with parents intervention on parent-infant closeness in NICU. *BMC Pediatrics, 21*(1), Article 28. https://doi.org/10.1186/s12887-020-02474-2

Head, L. M. (2014). The effect of kangaroo care on neurodevelopmental outcomes in preterm infants. *The Journal of Perinatal & Neonatal Nursing, 28*(4), 290–299. https://doi.org/10.1097/JPN.0000000000000062

Iwasa, K., & Ogawa, T. (2013). Rorschach texture responses are related to adult attachment via tactile imagery and emotion. *Rorschachiana, 34*(2), 115–136. https://doi.org/10.1027/1192-5604/a000045

Jack, R. E., & Schyns, P. G. (2015). The human face as a dynamic tool for social communication. *Current Biology, 25*(14), R621–R634. https://doi.org/10.1016/j.cub.2015.05.052

Jakubiak, B. K., & Feeney, B. C. (2017). Affectionate touch to promote relational, psychological, and physical well-being in adulthood: A theoretical model and review of the research. *Personality and Social Psychology Review, 21*(3), 228–252. https://doi.org/10.1177/1088868316650307

Jean, A. D. L., & Stack, D. M. (2012). Full-term and very-low-birth-weight preterm infants' self-regulating behaviours during a still-face interaction: Influences of maternal touch. *Infant Behaviour and Development, 35*(4), 779–791. https://doi.org/10.1016/j.infbeh.2012.07.023

Jean, A. D. L., Stack, D. M., & Fogel, A. (2009). A longitudinal investigation of maternal touching across the first 6 months of life: Age and context effects. *Infant Behaviour and Development, 32*(3), 344–349. https://doi.org/10.1016/j.infbeh.2009.04.005

Kirsch, L. P., Besharati, S., Papadaki, C., Crucianelli, L., Bertagnoli, S., Ward, N., Moro, V., Jenkinson, P. M., & Fotopoulou, A. (2020). Damage to the right insula disrupts the perception of affective touch. *eLife, 9.* https://doi.org/10.7554/eLife.47895

Kraus, J., Roman, R., Jurkovičová, L., Mareček, R., Mikl, M., Brázdil, M., & Frick, A. (2020). Social support modulates subjective and neural responses to sad mental imagery. *Behavioural Brain Research, 380*, Article 112433. https://doi.org/10.1016/j.bbr.2019.112433

Kreuder, A.-K., Scheele, D., Wassermann, L., Wollseifer, M., Stoffel-Wagner, B., Lee, M. R., Hennig, J., Maier, W., & Hurlemann, R. (2017). How the brain codes intimacy: The neurobiological substrates of romantic touch. *Human Brain Mapping, 38*(9), 4525–4534. https://doi.org/10.1002/hbm.23679

Leonard, J. A., Berkowitz, T., & Shusterman, A. (2014). The effect of friendly touch on delay-of-gratification in preschool children. *The Quarterly Journal of Experimental Psychology, 67*(11), 2123–2133. https://doi.org/10.1080/17470218.2014.907325

Liu, D., Diorio, J., Tannenbaum, B., Caldji, C., Francis, D., Freedman, A., Sharma, S., Pearson, D., Plotsky, P. M., & Meaney, M. J. (1997). Maternal care, hippocampal glucocorticoid receptors, and hypothalamic-pituitary-adrenal responses to stress. *Science, 277*(5332), 1659–1662. https://doi.org/10.1126/science.277.5332.1659

Löken, L. S., Wessberg, J., Morrison, I., McGlone, F., & Olausson, H. (2009). Coding of pleasant touch by unmyelinated afferents in humans. *Nature Neuroscience, 12*(5), 547–548. https://doi.org/10.1038/nn.2312

Longhi, E., Senna, I., Bolognini, N., Bulf, H., Tagliabue, P., Cassia, V. M., & Turati, C. (2015). Discrimination of biomechanically possible and impossible hand movements at birth. *Child Development, 86*(2), 632–641. https://doi.org/10.1111/cdev.12329

Mantis, I., Stack, D. M., Ng, L., Serbin, L. A., & Schwartzman, A. E. (2014). Mutual touch during mother-infant face-to-face still-face interactions: Influences of interaction period and infant birth status. *Infant Behaviour & Development, 37*(3), 258–267. https://doi.org/10.1016/j.infbeh.2014.04.005

McGlone, F., Wessberg, J., & Olausson, H. (2014). Discriminative and affective touch: Sensing and feeling. *Neuron, 82*(4), 737–755. https://doi.org/10.1016/j.neuron.2014.05.001

Meaney, M. J., & Szyf, M. (2005). Environmental programming of stress responses through DNA methylation: Life at the interface between a dynamic environment and a fixed genome. *Dialogues in Clinical Neuroscience, 7*(2), 103–123.

Mercuri, M., Stack, D. M., Trojan, S., Giusti, L., Morandi, F., Mantis, I., & Montirosso, R. (2019). Mothers' and fathers' early tactile contact behaviours during triadic and dyadic parent-infant interactions immediately after birth and at 3-months postpartum: Implications for early care behaviours and intervention. *Infant Behaviour and Development, 57*, Article 101347. https://doi.org/10.1016/j.infbeh.2019.101347

Moenter, A. (2020). Being in touch: The potential benefits and the use of attuned touch in psychotherapy for functional neurological symptoms (FNS). *European Journal of Trauma & Dissociation, 4*(3), Article 100161. https://doi.org/10.1016/j.ejtd.2020.100161

Montirosso, R., & McGlone, F. (2020). The body comes first. Embodied reparation and the co-creation of infant bodily-self. *Neuroscience and Biobehavioural Reviews, 113*, 77–87. https://doi.org/10.1016/j.neubiorev.2020.03.003

Montirosso, R., & Provenzi, L. (2015). Implications of epigenetics and stress regulation on research and developmental care of preterm infants. *Journal of Obstetric, Gynecologic, and Neonatal Nursing, 44*(2), 174–182. https://doi.org/10.1111/1552-6909.12559

Mörelius, E., Örtenstrand, A., Theodorsson, E., & Frostell, A. (2015). A randomised trial of continuous skin-to-skin contact after preterm birth and the effects on salivary cortisol, parental stress, depression, and breastfeeding. *Early Human Development, 91*(1), 63–70. https://doi.org/10.1016/j.earlhumdev.2014.12.005

Moszkowski, R. J., Stack, D. M., & Chiarella, S. S. (2009). Infant touch with gaze and affective behaviours during mother–infant still-face interactions: Co-occurrence and functions of touch. *Infant Behaviour & Development, 32*(4), 392–403. https://doi.org/10.1016/j.infbeh.2009.06.006

Müller-Oerlinghausen, B., & Eggart, M. (2021). Touch research – quo vadis? A plea for high-quality clinical trials. *Brain Sciences, 11*(1), Article 25. https://doi.org/10.3390/brainsci11010025

Novembre, G., Etzi, R., & Morrison, I. (2021). Hedonic responses to touch are modulated by the perceived attractiveness of the caresser. *Neuroscience, 464,* 79–89. https://doi.org/10.1016/j.neuroscience.2020.10.007

Olausson, H., Wessberg, J., Morrison, I., McGlone, F., & Vallbo, A. (2010). The neurophysiology of unmyelinated tactile afferents. *Neuroscience and Biobehavioural Reviews, 34*(2), 185–191. https://doi.org/10.1016/j.neubiorev.2008.09.011

Porges, S. W. (2007). The polyvagal perspective. *Biological Psychology, 74*(2), 116–143. https://doi.org/10.1016/j.biopsycho.2006.06.009

Provenzi, L., Brambilla, M., Scotto di Minico, G., Montirosso, R., & Borgatti, R. (2020). Maternal caregiving and DNA methylation in human infants and children: Systematic review. *Genes, Brain and Behaviour, 19*(3), Article e12616. https://doi.org/10.1111/gbb.12616

Provenzi, L., Giorda, R., Beri, S., & Montirosso, R. (2016). SLC6A4 methylation as an epigenetic marker of life adversity exposures in humans: A systematic review of literature. *Neuroscience and Biobehavioral Reviews, 71,* 7–20. https://doi.org/10.1016/j.neubiorev.2016.08.021

Provenzi, L., Lindstedt, J., De Coen, K., Gasparini, L., Peruzzo, D., Grumi, S., Arrigoni, F., & Ahlqvist-Björkroth, S. (2021). The paternal brain in action: A review of human fathers' fMRI brain responses to child-related stimuli. *Brain Sciences, 11*(6), Article 816. https://doi.org/10.3390/brainsci11060816

Provenzi, L., Rosa, E., Visintin, E., Mascheroni, E., Guida, E., Cavallini, A., & Montirosso, R. (2020). Understanding the role and function of maternal touch in children with neurodevelopmental disabilities. *Infant Behaviour and Development, 58,* Article 101420. https://doi.org/10.1016/j.infbeh.2020.101420

Rochat, P. (2021). Clinical pointers from developing self-awareness. *Developmental Medicine and Child Neurology, 63*(4), 382–386. https://doi.org/10.1111/dmcn.14767

Scher, M. S., Ludington-Hoe, S., Kaffashi, F., Johnson, M. W., Holditch-Davis, D., & Loparo, K. A. (2009). Neurophysiologic assessment of brain maturation after an 8-week trial of skin-to-skin contact on preterm infants. *Clinical Neurophysiology, 120*(10), 1812–1818. https://doi.org/10.1016/j.clinph.2009.08.004

Seidl, A., Tincoff, R., Baker, C., & Cristia, A. (2015). Why the body comes first: Effects of experimenter touch on infants' word finding. *Developmental Science, 18*(1), 155–164. https://doi.org/10.1111/desc.12182

Sharp, H., Pickles, A., Meaney, M., Marshall, K., Tibu, F., & Hill, J. (2012). Frequency of infant stroking reported by mothers moderates the effect of prenatal depression on infant behavioural and physiological outcomes. *PLoS One, 7*(10), Article e45446. https://doi.org/10.1371/journal.pone.0045446

Simpson, E. A., Maylott, S. E., Lazo, R. J., Leonard, K. A., Kaburu, S. S. K., Suomi, S. J., Paukner, A., & Ferrari, P. F. (2019). Social touch alters newborn monkey behaviour. *Infant Behaviour & Development, 57,* Article 101368. https://doi.org/10.1016/j.infbeh.2019.101368

Slater, R., Boyd, S., Meek, J., & Fitzgerald, M. (2006). Cortical pain responses in the infant brain. *Pain, 123*(3), Article 332. https://doi.org/10.1016/j.pain.2006.05.009

Stenzel, C. L., & Rupert, P. A. (2004). Psychologists' use of touch in individual psychotherapy. *Psychotherapy, 41*(3), 332–345. https://doi.org/10.1037/0033-3204.41.3.332

Stoll, B. J., Hansen, N. I., Bell, E. F., Shankaran, S., Laptook, A. R., Walsh, M. C., Hale, E. C., Newman, N. S., Schibler, K., Carlo, W. A., Kennedy, K. A., Poindexter, B. B., Finer, N. N., Ehrenkranz, R. A., Duara, S., Sánchez, P. J., O'Shea, T. M., Goldberg, R. N., Van Meurs, K. P., ..., & Higgins, R. D. (2010). Neonatal outcomes of extremely preterm infants from the NICHD Neonatal Research Network. *Pediatrics, 126*(3), 443–456. https://doi.org/10.1542/peds.2009-2959

Suvilehto, J. T., Glerean, E., Dunbar, R. I. M., Hari, R., & Nummenmaa, L. (2015). Topography of social touching depends on emotional bonds between humans. *Proceedings of the National Academy of Sciences of the United States of America, 112*(45), 13811–13816. https://doi.org/10.1073/pnas.1519231112

Tanaka, Y., Kanakogi, Y., Kawasaki, M., & Myowa, M. (2018). The integration of audio-tactile information is modulated by multimodal social interaction with physical contact in infancy. *Developmental Cognitive Neuroscience, 30*, 31–40. https://doi.org/10.1016/j.dcn.2017.12.001

Tanaka, Y., Kanakogi, Y., & Myowa, M. (2021). Social touch in mother–infant interaction affects infants' subsequent social engagement and object exploration. *Humanities and Social Sciences Communications, 8*(1). https://doi.org/10.1057/s41599-020-00642-4

Turati, C., Montirosso, R., Brenna, V., Ferrara, V., & Borgatti, R. (2011). A smile enhances 3-month-olds' recognition of an individual face. *Infancy, 16*(3), 306–317. https://doi.org/10.1111/j.1532-7078.2010.00047.x

Tuulari, J. J., Scheinin, N. M., Lehtola, S., Merisaari, H., Saunavaara, J., Parkkola, R., Sehlstedt, I., Karlsson, L., Karlsson, H., & Björnsdotter, M. (2019). Neural correlates of gentle skin stroking in early infancy. *Developmental Cognitive Neuroscience, 35*, 36–41. https://doi.org/10.1016/j.dcn.2017.10.004

Vindegaard, N., & Benros, M. E. (2020). COVID-19 pandemic and mental health consequences: Systematic review of the current evidence. *Brain, Behaviour, and Immunity, 89*, 531–542. https://doi.org/10.1016/j.bbi.2020.05.048

Walker, S. C., Trotter, P. D., Swaney, W. T., Marshall, A., & Mcglone, F. P. (2017). C-tactile afferents: Cutaneous mediators of oxytocin release during affiliative tactile interactions? *Neuropeptides, 64*, 27–38. https://doi.org/10.1016/j.npep.2017.01.001

Werbart, A. (2019). "The skin is the cradle of the soul": Didier Anzieu on the skin-ego, boundaries, and boundlessness. *Journal of the American Psychoanalytic Association, 67*(1), 37–58. https://doi.org/10.1177/0003065119829701

Westland, G. (2011). Physical touch in psychotherapy: Why are we not touching more? *Body Movement and Dance in Psychotherapy, 6*(1), 17–29. https://doi.org/10.1080/17432979.2010.508597

Westrup, B. (2007). Newborn Individualized Developmental Care and Assessment Program (NIDCAP)–family-centered developmentally supportive care. *Early Human Development, 83*(7), 443–449. https://doi.org/10.1016/j.earlhumdev.2007.03.006

History
Received October 18, 2021
Accepted November 10, 2021
Published online August 10, 2022

Conflict of Interest
The authors have none to declare.

Funding
The authors have none to declare.

ORCID
Livio Provenzi
ⓘhttps://orcid.org/0000-0001-7424-8744

Livio Provenzi
IRCCS Mondino Foundation
via Mondino 2
27100 Pavia
Italy
livio.provenzi@unipv.it

Summary

Since the seminal work of Freud, psychologists have been interested in the reciprocal connections between our body and our mind. Although visual stimuli have been a major topic in infant research and psychological science in general for decades, tactile dimensions of human social interactions are emerging as relevant source of information on human socio-emotional and socio-cognitive development. Recent advances at the intersection of psychology and social neuroscience are highlighting a specific neurophysiological underpinning, namely, the C-tactile fibers, which may help us understand how peripheral body interactions (i.e., social touch) can be embedded into our psychological development and functioning. C-tactile fibers are meant to be specifically responsive to gentle and affectionate social touch in humans. In other words, they may act as the neurophysiological substrate of our positive and nurturing socio-tactile interactions. In the present work, we describe the neurophysiological system that links the C-tactile fibers with specific brain regions, including the insula – a region of the brain that is involved in the early emergence of a child body image. Moreover, we provide evidence of the importance of social touch across development in typical and risk conditions and we highlight research and clinical implications for adults' emotional well-being and mental health.

Sommario

A partire dall'opera seminale di Freud, gli psicologi si sono interessati alle reciproche connessioni tra il nostro corpo e la nostra mente. Sebbene gli stimoli visivi siano stati per decenni un argomento di primario interesse nella ricerca infantile e nella scienza psicologica in generale, le dimensioni tattili delle interazioni sociali umane stanno emergendo come un'ulteriore fonte parimenti rilevante di informazioni sullo sviluppo socio-emotivo e socio-cognitivo umano. I recenti progressi al crocevia tra la psicologia e le neuroscienze sociali stanno mettendo in evidenza un supporto neurofisiologico specifico, vale a dire le fibre C-tattili, che possono aiutarci a capire come le interazioni corporee periferiche - cioè il contatto sociale - possono essere incorporate nel nostro sviluppo e funzionamento psicologico. Si pensa che le fibre C-tattili siano specificamente reattive al tocco sociale gentile e affettuoso negli umani. In altre parole, possono agire come substrato neurofisiologico delle nostre interazioni socio-tattili positive e associate a un senso di affiliazione. Nel presente lavoro, descriviamo il sistema neurofisiologico che collega le fibre C-tattili con specifiche regioni del cervello, inclusa l'insula, una regione del cervello coinvolta nell'emergere precoce dell'immagine corporea di un bambino. Inoltre, forniamo prove dell'importanza del contatto sociale attraverso lo sviluppo in condizioni tipiche e di rischio e mettiamo in evidenza la ricerca e le implicazioni cliniche per il benessere emotivo e la salute mentale degli adulti.

Résumé

Depuis les travaux fondateurs de Freud, les psychologues se sont intéressés aux connexions réciproques entre notre corps et notre esprit. Bien que les stimuli visuels soient un sujet majeur dans la recherche infantile et la science psychologique en général depuis des décennies, les dimensions tactiles des interactions sociales humaines apparaissent comme une source d'information pertinente sur le développement socio-émotionnel et socio-cognitif humain. Des avancées récentes à la croisée des chemins entre la psychologie et les neurosciences sociales mettent en évidence un fondement neurophysiologique spécifique, à savoir les fibres C-tactiles, qui peuvent nous aider à comprendre comment les interactions corporelles périphériques - c'est-à-dire le contact social - peuvent être intégrées dans notre développement et fonctionnement psychologiques. Les fibres C-tactiles sont conçues pour être spécifiquement sensibles au toucher social doux et affectueux chez les humains. En d'autres termes, ils peuvent agir comme le substrat neurophysiologique de nos interactions socio-tactiles positives et nourricières. Dans le présent travail, nous décrivons le système neurophysiologique qui relie les fibres C-tactiles à des régions cérébrales spécifiques, y compris l'insula - une région du cerveau impliquée dans l'émergence précoce d'une image corporelle de l'enfant. De plus, nous fournissons des preuves de l'importance du contact social dans le développement dans des conditions typiques et à risque et nous mettons en évidence la recherche et les implications cliniques pour le bien-être émotionnel et la santé mentale des adultes.

Resumen

Desde la obra fundamental de Freud, los psicólogos se han interesado por las conexiones recíprocas entre nuestro cuerpo y nuestra mente. Aunque los estímulos visuales han sido un tema importante en la investigación infantil y la ciencia psicológica en general durante décadas, las dimensiones táctiles de las interacciones sociales humanas están emergiendo como una fuente relevante de información sobre el desarrollo socioemocional y sociocognitivo humano. Los avances recientes en la encrucijada entre la psicología y la neurociencia social están destacando un sustento neurofisiológico específico, a saber, las fibras táctiles C, que pueden ayudarnos a comprender cómo las interacciones corporales periféricas, es decir, el contacto social, pueden integrarse en nuestro desarrollo y funcionamiento psicológico. Las fibras táctiles C están destinadas a responder específicamente al contacto social suave y afectuoso en los seres humanos. En otras palabras, pueden actuar como el sustrato neurofisiológico de nuestras interacciones socio-táctiles positivas y enriquecedoras. En el presente trabajo, describimos el sistema neurofisiológico que une las fibras táctiles C con regiones cerebrales específicas, incluida la ínsula, una región del cerebro que participa en la aparición temprana de una imagen corporal infantil. Además, proporcionamos evidencia de la importancia del contacto social en el desarrollo en condiciones típicas y de riesgo y destacamos la investigación y las implicaciones clínicas para el bienestar emocional y la salud mental de los adultos.

要約

フロイトの独創的な研究以来、心理学者は私たちの身体と心の相互関係に関心を寄せてきた。視覚的刺激は、数十年にわたり乳幼児研究および心理学一般の主要なトピックであったが、人間の社会的相互作用の触覚的側面が、人間の社会的情緒や社会的認知の発達に関する関連情報として注目されてきている。心理学と社会神経科学が融合した最近の研究では、C触覚線維はという特定の神経生理学的基盤が注目されており、これが身体周辺部の相互作用（すなわち、社会的接触）が、人の心理的発達や機能にどのように組み込まれるのかを理解するのに役立つと考えられる。C触覚線維は、人間の優しく愛情深い社会的接触に特異的に反応することを示している。つまり、C触覚線維は私たちの積極的な社会的触覚相互作用の神経生理学的基盤として機能している可能性がある。本研究では、C触覚線維と子どものボディイメージ形成に関わる島皮質など特定の脳領域とを結びつける神経生物学的システムを明らかにすることを目的としている。さらに、定型発達、リスク発達にわたる発達全体における社会的接触の重要性のエビデンスを示し、成人の感情的な幸福とメンタルヘルスに対する研究と臨床的意義を強調する。

Instructions to Authors

Rorschachiana is the scientific publication of the International Society for the Rorschach. The journal is interested in advancing theory and clinical applications of the Rorschach and other projective techniques, and research work that can enhance and promote projective methods.

***Rorschachiana* publishes the following types of articles:** Original Articles, Research Articles, and Case Studies.

Manuscript Submission: Manuscripts should be submitted online at
https://www.editorialmanager.com/ror
Detailed instructions to authors are provided at http://www.hgf.io/ror

Online Rights for Journal Articles: Guidelines on authors' rights to archive electronic version of their manuscripts online are given in the document "Guidelines on sharing and use of articles in Hogrefe journals" on the journal's web page at http://www.hgf.io/ror

September 2021